CARING FOR THE

PARKINSON
PATIENT

Golden Age Books
Perspective on Aging

Series Editor: Steven L. Mitchell

CARING FOR THE
PARKINSON
PATIENT

EDITED BY
J. THOMAS HUTTON, M.D., PH.D.
AND RAYE LYNNE DIPPEL, PH.D.

A PRACTICAL GUIDE

Golden Age Books

PROMETHEUS BOOKS
Buffalo, New York

Published 1989 by Prometheus Books
700 East Amherst Street, Buffalo, New York 14215

Library of Congress Cataloging-in-Publicaiton Data

Caring for the Parkinson patient: a practical guide/edited by J. Thomas Hutton and Raye Lynne Dippel.
     p.   cm.—(Golden age books)
    Includes bibliographical references.
    ISBN 0-87975-478-8 (cloth)—ISBN 0-87975-562-8—pbk.
    1. Parkinsonism—Patients—home care. 2. Parkinsonism—Patients—
Rehabilitation. 3. Parkinsonism—Patients—Medical care. 4. Self-
care, Health. I. Hutton, J. Thomas. II. Dippel, Raye Lynne.
III. Series.
RC382.C38   1989   89-10658
362.1'96833—dc20   CIP

Printed in the United States of America

Foreword

Michel Monnot
(author of *From Rage to Courage*)

The timeliness and usefulness of Dr. Hutton's and Dr. Dippel's new book is as much a credit to its assembled authors as it will be a mainstay in the caring program of Parkinsonian patients and caregivers. It addresses pertinent issues with such expertise that in reading it I could only exclaim: "Where were you, dear Dr. Hutton and your team, about ten years ago, when I and my contemporary Parkinsonians needed you so desperately? On that fateful day our respective neurologists delicately turned their heads away from us to announce: 'You, and you, and you, have Parkinson's disease'; and we were turned away without a shred of hope. We sat on the doctor's office steps and bawled our eyes out."

Today, in order "to ease the burden," newly diagnosed patients have a variety of coping mechanisms and strategies at their disposal: new drugs, support groups, enhanced surgical procedures, and the tantalizing successes of research that nurture the ever-growing hope "to find a cure."

Drs. Hutton and Dippel have edited a book that considers all these topics. It is a compendium of fourteen issue-directed chapters that give both caregiver and patient a global yet detailed guide for caring . . . and carrying on. Learn from these insights. Practice their suggestions and let them guide you to a fuller life.

Foreword

Frank L. Williams

(Director, The American Parkinson Disease Association)

As Executive Director of the American Parkinson Disease Association, I heartily endorse *Caring for the Parkinson Patient: A Practical Guide* and applaud the depth, understanding, and sensitivity with which Drs. Hutton and Dippel and their colleagues, address the physical and emotional problems endured by the Parkinsonian and the caregiver.

Not too many years ago, little information was available that could explain why the bodies of those with Parkinson's disease suddenly became frozen; why their vocal capacity had diminished to a whisper or why tremor made eating an almost impossible chore. Coping with Parkinson's disease is not and never will be easy. However, with greater knowledge and understanding of the disorder and its classic symptoms, coping can be made easier. This important new book provides the answers to many questions facing the newly diagnosed Parkinsonian as well as those who have suffered its burden for many years. This collection of essays constitutes a digest of clinical information that has emerged through scientific study and long-term evaluation, which will assist both the caregiver and the patient in their pursuit of a happier and healthier life for Parkinsonians as well as their spouses and family members.

Caring for the Parkinson Patient helps to "ease the burden" and details each phase of Parkinson's disease with the knowledge and skill that has become Dr. Hutton's trademark.

7

Preface

Exciting new research discoveries and dramatic advances in therapy for Parkinson's disease have occurred in recent years. Nevertheless, a person afflicted with this chronic neurological disorder still confronts the threat of reduced mobility and lessened psychological well-being. The practical problems presented by Parkinson's disease are many. The present volume is designed to provide relevant information for Parkinsonians, their families, and caregivers to aid in coping with this prevalent neurological disorder.

The volume begins with an overview of this medical disorder and describes principles of medical diagnosis and treatment. Dr. Henrik Kulmala follows with a description of the recent and exciting scientific research discoveries that may presage future improvements in therapy and the understanding of underlying causes. The experimental therapy of neurotransplanation is expertly handled by Dr. William Koller. A variety of practical approaches to make life with Parkinson's disease a bit easier are offered in Nelda Dippel's chapter, which covers nursing care. Although speech can be impaired by Parkinson's disease, the practical communication tips provided by Kathy Blakesley can improve speech performance. Maintaining mobility through physical therapy is covered in the chapter by Jim Carpenter. The serious complication of falls, with their attendant assault on self-esteem, is described in very practical terms by Carolyn Marshall. Inability to enjoy restful sleep is a source of irritation for many persons with Parkinson's disease. Useful approaches designed to cope with sleep disturbance are offered by Dr. Raye Lynne Dippel and Dr. J. Thomas Hutton. In separate chapters, Dr. Terry McMahon and Dr. Raye Lynne Dippel address the psychiatric aspects of Parkinson's disease and the depression that may be associated with the disorder. Dr. Jeffrey Elias and Dr. J. Thomas Hutton address cognitive changes. They approach their topic from a research and theoretical perspective. Although a single family member may have Parkinson's disease, the entire family is to some degree

9

affected by this disorder. The effect on family interaction is cogently described by Dr. Karen Boyd-Worley. The benefits and importance of community support systems are provided by Susan Imke and Dr. J. Thomas Hutton. Fred McGarrett and Dr. Raye Lynne Dippel round out the discussion of Parkinson's disease by offering a helpful guide for developing a successful support group from which members receive a constant flow of new information on therapy and services along with the benefits from ongoing mutual support.

The editors would like to express their appreciation to the contributors of this interdisciplinary volume. In addition, we thank our patients from whom we've gained both knowledge and inspiration. We also thank Mr. Steven L. Mitchell and the staff at Prometheus Books for their professional assistance. Finally, we thank our families for their understanding and support throughout the lengthy process of completing this volume.

J. Thomas Hutton, M.D., Ph.D.   Raye Lynne Dippel, Ph.D.

Contents

11

1

Diagnosis and Treatment

J. Thomas Hutton

OVERVIEW

What Is Parkinsonism?

Parkinsonism refers to a medical condition characterized by tremor, slow and reduced movements, and muscular stiffness. In the United States alone, approximately one million persons are estimated to suffer some form of Parkinsonism, the most common form of which is Parkinson's disease: a slow progressive brain disease of unknown cause affecting certain of the deeper structures (basal ganglia) in the brain. It is associated with the depletion of a brain chemical known as dopamine; this chemical loss tends to be focused particularly in a black pigmented area of the midbrain called the substantia nigra. The reduced dopamine brings about impaired communication between neurons of the substantia nigra and those of a nearby part of the brain known as the corpus striatum (the caudate and putaminal nuclei), resulting in the symptoms of Parkinson's disease (see figure 1).

Disorders that Resemble Parkinson's Disease

The symptoms of Parkinsonism are often drug-induced. Tranquilizing medications are the most common drugs that cause Parkinson-like symptoms.

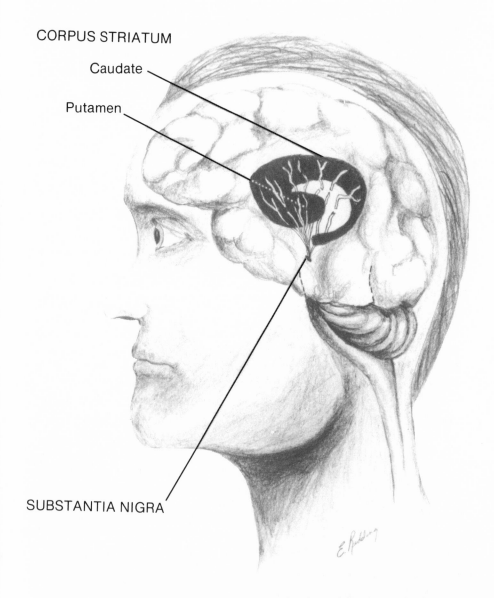

Figure 1. The substantia nigra is located in the midbrain and connects to the corpus striatum (caudate and putamen). The communication between these structures is mediated principally by the chemical messenger dopamine.

Such medications as haloperidol (Haldol), chlorpromazine (Thorazine), loxapine (Loxitane), trifluoroperazine (Stelazine), and fluphenazine (Prolixin) may give rise to clinical symptoms indistinguishable from Parkinson's disease. Reserpine, which may be used for high blood pressure or as a tranquilizing agent, also may give rise to Parkinsonism. This is not to suggest that all tranquilizing medications carry such a risk factor. Tranquilizers of the benzodiazepine class—such as diazepam (Valium), chlordiazepoxide (Librium), and alprazolam (Xanax)—do not cause symptoms of Parkinsonism.

Parkinsonism can also result from small strokes that, when they are diagnosed, can usually be traced to a preexisting high blood pressure condition. For a person who has suffered small strokes (or lacunes), slowness of movement and stiffness of the muscles may be present, in addition to general weakness or sensory loss. A careful neurological examination will usually differentiate this disorder from true Parkinson's disease. This so-called arteriosclerotic form of Parkinsonism does not respond well to the medications used to treat Parkinson's disease and is more likely to be associated with medication side effects.

Encephalitis (inflammation of the brain) may also give rise to Parkinsonism. A particular form of encephalitis swept the world in epidemic proportions between 1918 and 1925 leaving many persons with Parkinsonism. The postencephalitis form of Parkinsonism damaged the basal ganglia of the brain, but is rarely seen today. Tremor was unusual with this form of Parkinsonism.

In 1985, several instances of Parkinsonism resulted from a street drug contaminated with a chemical known as MPTP. This extremely toxic agent selectively damages the same areas that are injured in Parkinson's disease and gives rise to the same symptoms. The victims respond favorably to levodopa, which is the principal medication used to treat Parkinsonian patients. Although the discovery of MPTP was a tragedy to those afflicted, it did open a promising new area for Parkinson's disease research (see chapter 2).

Another neurological disorder that has at times been mistaken for Parkinson's disease is essential or familial tremor. In this disorder, the hand tremor is faster and finer than that of Parkinson's disease and is most bothersome when patients attempt to use their hands. In contrast, Parkinsonian tremor is slower, more coarse, and most obvious when the hands are at rest. A person with essential or familial tremor does not have muscular rigidity or slowness of movements as do Parkinsonians. Essential tremor occurs sporadically, whereas the familial tremor runs in families, with approximately half the offspring developing it at some time during their lives.

Progressive supranuclear palsy has been called a "kissing cousin" of Parkinson's disease, though it is much less frequent. It, too, is a progressive neurological disease that adversely affects movement, while affecting balance earlier and more severely than with Parkinson's disease. The muscular stiffness is primarily of the neck and back muscles, unlike Parkinson's disease in which extremity stiffness is observed. The diagnosis of supranuclear palsy also requires that the patient's gaze be impaired, which typically consists of an inability to elevate or lower the eyes. Memory problems are often a prominent aspect of this progressive neurological disease.

DIAGNOSIS OF PARKINSON'S DISEASE

Clinical Signs of Parkinson's Disease

As in the time of James Parkinson (1755–1824), Parkinson's disease remains a diagnosis that is established by neurological examination. Such an exam may often be sufficient to identify and exclude the other disorders just described, any of which could be mistaken for Parkinson's disease. At the present time, no readily available laboratory test exists that will confirm the diagnosis of Parkinson's disease, although the computer assisted tomagraphy (CAT) scan and the magnetic resonance imaging (MRI) scan can rule out small strokes or tumors as causes of the Parkinsonism.

The clinical diagnosis of Parkinson's disease is made by a neurologist when three basic components are observed: a slow resting tremor, a particular form of muscular rigidity referred to as cogwheeling (which produces jerking movements), and slow or significantly reduced movement (bradykinesia). The tremor is four to five cycles per second and most commonly observed in the hands. The tremor has been described as a pill-rolling type, reminiscent of pharmacists of yesteryear who made pills by rolling them between their thumbs and fingers. Tremor may also be seen in the jaw and in lower extremities. The muscular rigidity is usually identified by the examiner as he moves the extremities back and forth while feeling for regular jerks as if a cogwheel were in the extremity. The bradykinesia may be of a general type in which the person lacks the usual minor changes in position and moves slowly, or it may be noted when the person attempts rapid fine movements of the hands or feet, such as tapping the heel or opening and closing the hands.

In addition to these three cardinal signs of Parkinson's disease, a number of minor signs exist. These include changes in speech, difficulty in swallowing, the presence of drooling, a noticeably stooped posture, a lack of arm swing when walking, a shuffling gait, loss of balance, blank staring facial expression (mask-like face), constipation, difficulty with bladder control, sexual dysfunction, and dandruff (seborrheic dermatitis). The speech pattern of a Parkinsonian is that of a muffled monotone. The volume of the speech is reduced and at times may be difficult to understand. Swallowing may also be impaired with aspiration (sucking of air) occurring into the windpipe. Drooling, referred to as sialorrhea, results from lack of automatic swallowing and is aggravated by the stooped posture of those with Parkinson's disease. The lack of associated arm swing during walking represents a loss of an automatic (involuntary) movement that typically occurs when the basal ganglia portion of the brain is not functioning properly. The balance problems result from a loss of the patient's normal ability to correct changes in posture (his or her righting reflexes) and from the feet "freezing," both of which may result in serious falls. For those who have lost these righting reflexes, a slight shove may find them completely unable to regain balance. Walking consists typically of short, shuffling steps. The patient may show propulsive or retropulsive gait in which an attempt is being made to keep the feet centered beneath the body to avoid falling. Constipation, poor bladder control, and impotence point to involvement of the autonomic nervous system with Parkinson's disease.

By convention, Parkinson's disease is diagnosed when at least two of the three major signs are present, or when one major sign and at least two minor signs are identified. Few patients ever develop all the signs of the disease, and substantial variation in the symptoms are often observed. Approximately one-fifth of those with Parkinson's disease never develop tremor, so that particular component is not a requirement for the diagnosis.

Parkinson's Disease Symptoms

slow, resting tremor
muscular rigidity (cogwheeling)
bradykinesia (slowness of movement)
poor balance
disturbance in gait (propulsive or retropulsive)
"freezing" (feet immobilized suddenly)
stooped posture
blank facial expression

difficulty swallowing
reduced volume and clarity of speech
sialorrhea (drooling)
seborrheic dermatitis (dandruff)
bladder control problems
constipation
sexual dysfunction
mood changes
sleep disturbance

Stages of Parkinson's Disease

Parkinson's disease is usually a slow, progressive disorder. A variety of scales have been developed to describe its severity. One commonly used clinical scale is that developed by Hoehn and Yahr, which divides the disease into five stages:

Stage I—Signs of Parkinson's disease strictly one-sided, affecting one side of the body only

Stage II—Signs of Parkinson's disease are bilateral but balance is not impaired

Stage III—Signs of Parkinson's disease are bilateral and balance is impaired

Stage IV—Parkinson's disease is functionally disabling

Stage V—Patient is confined to bed or a wheelchair

Progression through the stages of Parkinson's disease is highly variable. In rare instances a person may progress to stage IV or V in as little as five years, but more typically a patient may have Parkinson's disease for fifteen to twenty years before entering the severest stages. The staging of the disease also does not take into account the frequently seen clinical fluctuations. For example, an advanced Parkinsonian patient may be totally bedridden (Stage V) prior to a delayed dose of levodopa, but once the medication has taken effect the patient may improve to stage II or III.

MEDICATIONS FOR PARKINSON'S DISEASE

Principles of Drug Therapy

The goal of treating Parkinson's disease with a drug regimen is to reduce functional disability. For that reason it is important that the treating physician have an adequate knowledge of how the disease is affecting the life of each patient individually. A favorable balance is sought between improved motor performance and the side effects from medications. For example, a surgeon, a seamstress, or a typist will have more need to maintain tight control of the disease and will likely risk more medication side effects than would, say, an inactive or retired person. A good general rule of treatment is to improve everyday activity, not to eradicate every sign of Parkinsonism. With the exception of the first few years of levodopa treatment, it is usually impractical to mask completely the signs of the disease. Attempts to do so are fraught with increased risks of medication side effects.

A person with Parkinson's disease who is well versed in the goals and the possible adverse aspects of treatment, and who understands the expected course of the disorder, can greatly enhance the therapeutic outcome. The treating physician, who is often a neurologist, will have knowledge about which aspects of the disease are likely to improve with a given medication and what side effects are most likely to occur. An awareness of the expected progression of the disease is also important: too often patients incorrectly assume that worsening motor function is a result of ineffective medication rather than a sign identifying the changing nature of their disease. An evolving clinical picture requires periodic checkups and dosage readjustments.

Good and open communication between patient and treating physician is important. Patients bring to this relationship knowledge about the impact that the disease has had on their lives and a set of values that speak to the degree of risk and disability that can be tolerated. For their part, the physicians bring medical and scientific knowledge about the disease and a general understanding how other patients in similar circumstances have responded. The doctor/patient relationship is in a very real sense á contract requiring both to do their best to assure the most favorable outcome.

Patients who are knowledgeable about Parkinson's disease and have a good grasp of the symptoms, provide the possibility of limited flexible dosage schedules. From time to time these individuals may need increased medication: for example, prior to physical exertion or just before making a public appearance. I have found it useful to provide dosage flexibility for such persons in order to tailor the drug therapy to their needs. On the other hand, I have had some referral patients who ostensibly were unable to tolerate any anti-Parkinsonian medications. In these instances, invariably the person had failed to recognize that the "side effects" were in fact the signs of the disease itself. Dosage flexibility is only practical with a well-informed patient. Except for emergency situations, it is desirable for the patient to check with the doctor prior to discontinuing medications.

Anticholinergic Agents (tremor medications)

The first effective treatment for Parkinson's disease was tincture of belladonna (atropine and hyoscine) and was introduced in the nineteenth century by the famous French neurologist Jean Martin Charcot (1825-1893). A large number of other anticholinergic and antihistaminic medications were introduced during the 1940s and 1950s. These agents are most useful for the treatment of tremor. Since tremor is frequently the first sign of Parkinson's disease, it is not at all surprising that the anticholinergic and antihistaminic agents are often the first medications used in the treatment process (see table 1, p. 24). The anticholinergic agents also dry the mouth and may therefore prove useful in treating drooling. Unfortunately this class of medication has little or no positive effect on rigidity, slowness of movement, or other features of Parkinson's disease. The anticholinergic agents are of value in treating drug-induced Parkinsonism and post-encephalitic Parkinsonism.

A time honored, if slightly outmoded clinical concept, describes an imbalance between the cholinergic system and the dopaminergic system in the brains of Parkinsonians. This concept suggests that the symptoms of the disease may be improved either by increasing the amount of dopamine in the brain or by reducing the amount of acetylcholine (see figure 2, p. 21). The anticholinergic medications interfere with brain acetylcholine transmission and are believed to create a better balance between these two principal brain chemicals. Those anticholinergic agents still commonly in use include trihexyphenidyl (Artane), benzotropine (Cogentin), biperiden (Akineton), and procyclidine (Kemadrin).

Anticholinergic medications may give rise to side effects: for example, constipation and difficulty with emptying the bladder may result. Bladder problems and constipation are fairly common among Parkinsonian patients in any case, but these conditions can be further aggravated if anticholinergic

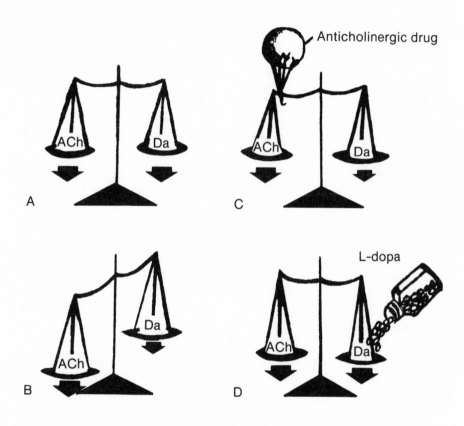

Figure 2. This figure demonstrates the balances between acetylcholine (ACh) and dopamine (Da) for normal and parkinsonian states. Panel A demonstrates the normal balance between acetylcholine and dopamine in normal, healthy persons. In B, which represents Parkinson's disease, the deficiency of dopamine is represented by an imbalance in favor of acetylcholine. Panel C represents restoration of this balance by an anticholinergic drug, which effectively reduces the effect of brain acetylcholine. Panel D represents an alternative therapeutic strategy of restoring the balance by providing levodopa, which is converted to dopamine, thereby increasing brain dopamine levels.

agents are part of the treatment. Blurring of vision and confusion may result from the anticholinergic effect on both the eye and the brain. Anticholinergic agents also impede sweating, which could lead to heat exhaustion for patients in hot climates or during the summer months. On the other hand, some Parkinsons patients experience excessive and abnormal sweating, which may be reduced by the anticholinergic medications.

Antihistamines

Antihistamines are a category of medications closely related to anticholinergics. It may be that the pharmacologic benefits of the antihistaminic agents result from anticholinergic properties, so that the antihistamines are generally considered along with the anticholinergic agents. The anti-Parkinsonian effects of the antihistamine medication is clearly unrelated to their effects on histamine.

Diphenhydramine (Benadryl) is an over-the-counter agent that is used particularly for the treatment of tremor. Chlorphenoxamine (Phenoxene) is an effective antitremor agent. These agents have less risk of causing or aggravating bladder and bowel problems, but may give rise to drowsiness, especially in the first few weeks of use.

Amantadine (Symmetrel)

Amantadine is frequently the initial treatment for Parkinson's disease, especially if slowness of movement or rigidity are the principal symptoms. It is generally well tolerated and acts clinically like a weak form of levodopa. The precise mechanism of action is unknown. It may exert its anti-Parkinsonian effect by increasing the release of dopamine stored in the brain. Amantadine does have a beneficial effect on rigidity, slowness of movement, and tremor.

The discovery of the anti-Parkinsonian effect of amantadine was serendipitous. Dr. Schwab learned from a patient who had been prescribed amantadine for influenza that her Parkinson's disease was helped. Dr. Schwab confirmed this observation: patients felt better and looked better when taking amantadine. This agent is now commonly used for mild and moderate forms of the disease.

Some experts believe that the wholesome effects of amantadine may be short lived. Others believe that the effect is ongoing, yet the progression of the disease after several months requires the physician to substitute or add a stronger medication. Whether or not the effects of amantadine are ephemeral, discontinuation of the medication may be associated with a substantial increase in Parkinsonian symptoms. Restarting the medication will usually reestablish control at the level that was present prior to discontinuance. If amantadine is to be discontinued, it is best to taper the dosage downward prior to discontinuing.

Visual hallucinations are a disturbing side effect of amantadine; they are observed particularly in advanced Parkinson's disease. The hallucinations frequently take the form of nonthreatening people or animals and may be very realistic. This adverse effect will go away when the medication is discontinued. Livido reticularis is a purplish skin mottling of the legs that may result from treatment with amantadine. This skin reaction is not serious but usually prompts discontinuation of the medication. Other possible side effects include congestive heart failure, lightheadedness or faintness upon standing, and ankle swelling. Visual blurring, constipation, and difficulty emptying the bladder may also occur as side effects of amantadine.

Levodopa (Sinemet, Madopar)

The introduction of levodopa (also called L-Dopa) in the mid-1960s for the treatment of Parkinson's disease followed the important discovery that dopamine was reduced in certain brain structures in Parkinsonians. Replacement therapy with levodopa, which is converted in the body to dopamine, brought about many dramatic clinical improvements. Levodopa continues to be the most widely used agent in treatment regimens and is effective at all stages of the disease. Typically, levodopa therapy is begun when muscular rigidity or slowness of movement start to impair everyday performance significantly. This is a highly effective treatment for the symptoms and signs of Parkinson's disease, yet neither levodopa nor any other anti-Parkinsonian agent has yet to affect a slowing of the underlying disease.

To prevent rapid breakdown of levodopa in the body, the drug is combined with either carbidopa or benserazide. Carbidopa/levodopa (Sinemet) is marketed through North America while benserazide/levodopa (Madopar) is marketed throughout Europe. By using either carbidopa or benserazide as blocking agents to prevent breakdown of levodopa before it reaches the brain, the total required amount of levodopa is reduced by 80 to 90 percent.

When a person with Parkinson's disease starts treatment with Sinemet or Madopar, the effects are typically dramatic. The bradykinesia (slowed

TABLE 1

MEDICATIONS COMMONLY USED IN THE TREATMENT OF PARKINSON'S DISEASE

MEDICATION	STAGE	USUAL DOSAGE RANGE	BENEFITS	MAIN SIDE EFFECTS
Anticholinergics:				
Trihexyphenidyl (Artane)	mild and moderate	2-20 mg/day	Reduces tremor and drooling	Mental changes
Benzotropine (Cogentin)	mild and moderate	0.5-6 mg/day	" "	Constipation
Biperiden (Adineton)	mild and moderate	2 mg/day	Reduces rigidity, especially in drug-induced PD	Difficulty with emptying bladder
Procyclidene (Kemadrin)	mild and moderate	2.5-15 mg/day	" "	Dry mouth
Antihistaminics:				
Diphenhydramine (Benadryl)	mild and moderate	25-200 mg/day	Reduces tremor, mildly sedating	Drowsiness
Chlorphenoxamine (Phenoxene)	mild and moderate	50-300 mg/day	" "	" "
Amantadine (Symmetrel)	mild and moderate	100-300 mg/day	Helps all aspects	Visual hallucinations, Confusion, Mottling of skin, Dizziness on standing
Carbidopa (A) / Levodopa (B) (Sinemet)	all stages	75-150 mg/day (A) 75-1000 mg/day (B)	Helps all aspects " "	Nausea, Involuntary movements, Confusion, Dizziness on standing
Bromocriptine (Parlodel)	all stages	1.25-20 mg/day	Helps all aspects	Confusion, Dizziness on standing, Nausea

or reduced movement), rigidity, and tremor are greatly improved to the extent that the person may be almost unaware of Parkinsonian symptoms. This so-called levodopa honeymoon usually lasts from two to five years. During this period of time, the patient usually does not feel any wearing off of the medication. Nevertheless, many Parkinsonians eventually begin to experience the wearing-off phenomenon or "end of dose" failure.

Wearing-off phenomenon may occur subtly: for example, when a person awakens in the morning and finds that the symptoms of the disease are particularly prominent. The patient may also experience the return of symptoms prior to the next scheduled dose of Sinemet. At this point in the treatment the patient can usually sense when the medication "kicks in," and becomes acutely aware of the need to take the medication regularly. The approach when treating the wearing-off phenomenon, or the even more abrupt rapid swings of on/off syndrome, consists of taking doses of Sinemet at more frequent intervals and often in smaller quantities.

The scientific understanding of wearing-off phenomenon and on/off syndrome is incomplete. The wearing-off phenomenon probably results from reduced storage of dopamine throughout the basal ganglia so that controlling the signs of the disease requires a fairly stable level of levodopa in the bloodstream. Unfortunately the blood level of levodopa is short-lived, lasting only a few hours, which requires either frequent dosing or adding another agent such as bromocriptine (Parlodel).

Another therapeutic approach to reducing motor fluctuations or wearing-off phenomenon springs from the observation that levodopa, when infused intravenously at a constant rate, will largely stop the motor fluctuations. The approach that has been tried consists of a controlled release tablet of carbidopa/levodopa (Sinemet CR) or benserazide/levodopa capsule (Madopar-HBS). The Sinemet CR, which is the better tested of the two agents, has been shown to reduce the need for frequent doses of medication and to improve control of Parkinson's disease as compared to standard Sinemet. Sinemet CR has been tested in multicenter trials and the results have been sent to the U.S. Food and Drug Administration for review. It is likely that Sinemet CR will be available for prescription usage by late 1989 or early 1990.

Although levodopa is the drug of choice for most Parkinsonians, it is not without side effects. When beginning the medication, it is best to start with small doses and build up over a period of several weeks. A positive effect will usually be seen in four to five days, but the complete effect may take several weeks. The slowly increased dosage will also limit the initial nausea—a frequent patient complaint. Occasionally vomiting occurs but it is rarely so severe as to prevent continued use of the medication. When beginning levodopa it is best to take it with food. Later, as tolerance is developed and more complete absorption is needed, the drug may be taken on an empty stomach or with a light nonprotein snack. (Dietary considerations will be discussed in more detail in this chapter and in chapter 4.)

With long-term use of levodopa, drug-induced abnormal movements may occur (dyskinesias). These movements may consist of mouth or tongue movements, or quick, nonpurposeful movements of the extremities; at times, writhing movements or fixed abnormal postures of the hands or feet may occur. These drug-induced dyskinesias usually occur when the levodopa in the bloodstream is at its maximum (on dystonia), although occasionally they occur when the drug level is at its minimum in the blood (off dystonia). Dyskinesias are usually seen in the context of advanced disease, suggesting that the underlying brain substrate is important in the evolution of this side effect. In addition, the long-term effects of levodopa bring about a change in the dopamine receptors in the brain, which may be involved in the evolution of dyskinesias.

Mental confusion and hallucinations pose a growing problem not only for the Parkinsonian patient but for the treating physician as well. In 1817, when James Parkinson originally described the disorder now bearing his name, he described the mental aspects of the disease as "the senses and intellect being uninjured." It is likely that prior to the advent of levodopa, persons with Parkinson's disease did not survive long enough for Parkinsonian dementia to occur. In addition, it is now well recognized that most of the anti-Parkinsonian agents may give rise to confusion disorders. This aspect of Parkinsonism is particularly perplexing to treat. As a general rule, if a state of confusion is experienced, all anti-Parkinsonian medications are discontinued with the exception of minimal doses of levodopa. The relative benefits of the drug must be weighed against its side effects. At times a drug holiday may be tried to determine if the confusion disorder is indeed the result of medication. Drug holidays, nevertheless, are not without significant risk of severe immobility with aspiration pneumonia and pulmonary emboli.

Lightheadedness and fainting can be side effects of levodopa. Upon arising quickly, the blood may rush to the legs, thus depriving the brain of adequate blood supply. Although this may occur in patients who are not treated with levodopa, it is often worsened by the medication. Typically this is not so severe as to alter therapy, but at times it may require the wearing of elastic stockings, or if necessary, discontinuing levodopa.

When taking levodopa, it is essential that monoamine oxidase inhibitors not be taken. The so-called MAO inhibitors (such as Parnate, Eutonyl, Furoxone, Marplan, and Nardil) are rarely prescribed today, but for a period of time they were used to treat depression. Such a combination has the potential to cause severe elevations in blood pressure and pulse rate. Alpha methyl dopa (Aldomet), which is used to treat high blood pressure, should not be prescribed in combination with levodopa: it reduces the effect of levodopa much like the major tranquilizers that were described earlier.

Bromocriptine (Parlodel)

Bromocriptine is termed a dopamine receptor agonist agent. In contrast to levodopa, which is converted to dopamine in the substantia nigra that secondarily stimulates the corpus striatum (caudate and putaminal nuclei), a dopamine agonist agent directly stimulates the dopamine receptors in the corpus striatum. The agonist agent in effect fools the corpus striatum into accepting it as dopamine. The agonist agent now in widespread use for the treatment of Parkinson's disease is bromocriptine (Parlodel). Other dopamine receptor agonist agents have been developed, tested, and may be released in the not-too-distant future.

Bromocriptine is most effective in the early to middle phases of the disease, though it is usually reserved for the middle stages. Bromocriptine is almost as effective as levodopa in treating the bradykinesia, muscular stiffness, and tremor, but most effective when used in combination with levodopa. Bromocriptine needs to be started in low doses, then gradually increased over a period of several months to lessen the risk of side effects. Though patience is required to use this medicine, the recipient is rewarded with improved motor function and some theoretical advantages.

The addition of bromocriptine to levodopa will allow smaller amounts of the latter to be used. This may be of some benefit in forestalling the onset of motor fluctuations. Bromocriptine may also be of benefit in smoothing out the daily course of motor fluctuations seen with levodopa-treated advanced Parkinson's disease. Many experienced neurologists now tend to use bromocriptine earlier in the course of the disease, but they also use it at lower doses (10 to 20 milligrams total daily dosage) than was originally recommended.

Bromocriptine has significant potential side effects. One of the most disturbing is confusion, which has been observed in nearly half the patients who use this therapy but is most prominent in patients with advanced disease. In my experience, confusion is much less likely when the agent is used in the early stages of Parkinson's disease and when used in younger patients. The severity of the confusion episode is greater than that associated with levodopa, amantadine, or the anticholinergics. Whereas a mild dementia may occur with Parkinson's disease, caution is advised when using bromocriptine for these patients. The drug-induced confusion disorder subsides over several days when the medication is discontinued. Nausea, vomiting, and lightheadedness are also side effects of bromocriptine. Dyskinesias have been described but are less common with bromocriptine than with levodopa.

Beta Blockers

Propranolol (Inderal) and nadolol (Corgard) are effective medications for the treatment of essential tremor and familial tremor. These agents are particularly beneficial for tremor of the hand, and to a lesser extent for those of the head and voice. For a long time it was believed that beta blockers were of no benefit in the treatment of Parkinson's disease. Recently these agents have been reevaluated and some benefits noted. In addition to having a slow tremor of the hands when at rest, some patients also have a rapid component of the tremor when the hands are suspended in front of them or when the hands are being used. This more rapid tremor is characteristic of essential (familial) tremor and may respond to the beta blockers.

Antidepressant Medications

Depression occurs in 20 to 40 percent of Parkinsonians, though in most cases it is mild. The origin of the depression results from Parkinson-related brain chemical changes, although psychological reactions to the chronic illness also play a part (see chapter 10).

Commonly used antidepressant medications include amitriptyline (Elavil), imipramine (Tofranil), doxepin (Sinequan), and nortriptyline (Pamelor). Antidepressant effects may not be realized for one to three weeks. All of these medications can cause drying of the mouth, increased constipation, and difficulty emptying the bladder.

Deprenyl (Jumex, Eldepryl)

Deprenyl is a medication currently being investigated in the United States but available in Europe for many years. Eldepryl has recently been released by the U.S. Food and Drug Administration for treatment of Parkinson's disease. The potent Parkinsonian effects of the neurotoxin MPTP can be prevented in animals by pretreating with deprenyl. This has led some to speculate that the progress of Parkinson's disease in humans may be favorably altered with ongoing deprenyl treatment. At the present time, ongoing research sponsored by the National Institutes of Health (USA) is investigating this medication in a large mulitcenter study.

Vitamin E

In recent years vitamin E (alpha tocopherol) has been discussed as a possible treatment. It is also being tested in the ongoing study of deprenyl to determine if the antioxidant effects of vitamin E may slow the progression of Parkinson's disease. Treatment with levodopa creates metabolic by-products in the brain that are oxidants and may hasten new symptoms. Vitamin E, which is an antioxidant, is designed to "sponge up" these potentially harmful by-products of levodopa therapy.

OTHER THERAPEUTIC APPROACHES

Exercise

Exercise plays a valuable role in the overall treatment plan. A regular program of exercise assists in maintaining muscle flexibility and will even reduce the need for medication. Stretching exercises are particularly beneficial given the increased muscular rigidity found in Parkinsonian patients. Consultation with a physical therapist can be useful to define an appropriate group of exercises that may be continued at home (see chapter 6).

Diet

Vitamin B_6 is known to inhibit the effectiveness of levodopa. This effect is seen only when levodopa is taken without an inhibitor, so that no particular concern exists when a Parkinsonian patient is taking either Sinemet or Madopar. Nevertheless, if levodopa is being taken in the form of Larodopa, then multiple vitamins containing vitamin B_6 should be avoided. Should vitamin supplements be desired, then a vitamin preparation without B_6 should be prescribed (such as Larobec).

In general, changes in diet have little effect on Parkinson's disease.

TABLE 2

PROTEIN REDISTRIBUTION DIET FOR PARKINSONIANS*

DAYTIME (PRIOR TO 5:00 P.M.)	EVENING MEAL
An unrestricted quantity of the following foods can be consumed [less than 10 gms. (grams) of protein]:	Meal should contain Recommended Daily Allowance for individual's age at ideal weight (approximately 30-50 gms. after 10 gms. consumed during day.)

Fluids: Coffee, tea, soda (nondiet), all fruit and vegetable juices, water, nondairy liquid creamers (e.g., Polyrich).

Fruits: All fresh and dried fruits.

Vegetables: All green and yellow vegetables (lettuce, onions, cucumbers, cauliflower, broccoli, squash, carrots, etc.); potatoes (skinless) cooked any way, including french fries.

Breads &   Certain cereals that are low in protein (Rainbow Brite, Rice Krispies,
Cereals: and Rice Chex—should contain 2 gm. or less protein per serving).

Graham crackers, melba toast, fried onion rings, toaster pastries.

Desserts: Italian ice, sherbet

Condiments: Oil, vinegar, margarine, butter, herbs, spices, sugar, honey, jellies and jams, pickles, hard candies, mints, powdered nondairy creamers.

FOODS TO AVOID BEFORE 5:00 P.M.:

Meat, meat products, fish, egg whites (yolk contains no protein), gelatin, dairy products (milk, sour cream, cheeses, yogurt, cottage cheese, ice cream); legumes such as kidney beans, lima beans, soy or pinto beans; nuts, peanut butter, chocolate, cookies, cakes, pastry, or pizza.

*Adapted from "Influence on Dietary Protein on Motor Fluctuations in Parkinson's Disease," by Jonathan H. Pincus, M.D., and Kathryn Barry, M.S.N., R.N.; *Archives of Neurology*, 44 (1987):270–272.

At times, however, in advanced stages of the disease, protein may impair the transport of levodopa to the brain. In such instances in which Parkinsonians tend to go "off" following a protein meal, a protein redistribution diet may prove helpful. The concept of protein redistribution is not to decrease the overall amount of protein in the diet, but rather to redistribute dietary protein to a time when the patient is likely to be sedentary or asleep. Typically, protein redistribution moves the protein to the evening meal, while breakfast and lunch are high in carbohydrates (see table 2, p. 30).

At times, when advanced Parkinsonians are having dyskinesias, ingestion of a protein snack may be of benefit; by impairing levodopa transport it thus diminishes the levodopa-induced dyskinesias. Such a protein snack may also be of some benefit in counteracting levodopa-induced vivid dreaming and nightmares.

Diets high in fiber and fruit may also help to reduce or avoid constipation. (For additional dietary information see chapter 4.)

SUPPORT ACTIVITIES

Parkinson's disease can be frightening for both the patient and the family. Access to a variety of support activities can assist those afflicted and their families to adjust to this chronic disease. The treating physician may be able to provide answers to many questions, and can also offer referrals to a variety of health care professionals for additional needs such as long-term counseling, physical therapy, occupational therapy, speech therapy, social services, dietary consultation, and support groups. All of these areas are discussed in the chapters that follow.

SUGGESTED READING

Duvoisin, Roger C. *Parkinson's Disease: A Guide for Patient and Family.* New York: Raven Press, 1985.

Lieberman, A. N.; G. Gopinathan; A. Neophytides; and M. Goldstein. *Parkinson's Disease Handbook.* American Parkinson Disease Association, 1989.

Pincus, Jonathan H., and Kathryn Barry. "Influence of Dietary Protein on Motor Fluctuations in Parkinson's Disease." *Archives of Neurology* 44 (1978): 270–272.

2

Parkinson's Disease Research

Henrik K. Kulmala

INTRODUCTION

Research on Parkinson's disease is an active area whose scope ranges from basic studies on the brain to clinical studies of drugs to control the symptoms, and potential ways to "cure" the disorder, including brain transplants. I will focus on studies concerning the cause, the diagnosis, the treatment, and the development of animal models of Parkinson's disease. To understand the research it is necessary to have some idea of the brain systems involved.

Parkinson's disease is caused when a loss of the chemical dopamine occurs in the brain. Dopamine is called a neurotransmitter because it is one of the chemicals that the brain cells (neurons) use to send messages to other neurons. The act of neurotransmission consists of the release of a chemical, such as dopamine, from a neuron in response to an electrical impulse in that neuron. Dopamine then moves across a small gap (called a synapse) between neurons, where it binds to molecules called receptors on other neurons. Put in more graphic terms, dopamine is the key that unlocks the receptor neurons. Placing the "key" into the "lock" opens or closes a "door" causing or stopping electrical activity in the next neuron. The loss of dopamine in Parkinson's disease stops such neurotransmission and brings about the symptoms of the disorder.

The brain is a very complex organ that uses many neurotransmitters to function. Dopamine is not found throughout the brain; rather, it is localized in a few specific cell clusters. In Parkinson's disease, it is the loss of one of these brain cell clusters (the substantia nigra) that causes the disease. It was known for many years that the substania nigra was involved in the disease, long before the discovery of dopamine as a neurotransmitter. The substantia nigra (literally black substance) is a cluster of neurons that appears black because of a chemical called melanin, which is related to dopamine. The loss of these black cells was easily detected in autopsies.

The substantia nigra dopamine neurons send projections—long fibers called axons—to another brain area called the striatum, where they influence other cells. (Please refer to Dr. Hutton's figure 1, p. 14.) Thus, Parkinsons's disease is caused by a loss of the dopamine-containing nigrostriatal pathway in the brain. Alternatively, those who manifest the disease experience a lack of balance in the striatum between dopamine and another neurotransmitter called acetylcholine. The treatment of Parkinson's disease consists of an attempt to restore this balance, either by adding dopamine or by subtracting the effects of acetylcholine.

To understand Parkinson's disease research, a simple analogy is needed to explain how the brain works. Each brain cell can be thought of as a wire, connecting one brain area with another. Actually, there are brain cells called glia whose functions do not include neurotransmission, but keep other cells functioning by providing nutrients and also insulating neurons. These glia are much less studied but are very important in maintaining brain function. The neurons, or "wires," connect with other "wires" through a massive switching system. At the start of any such "wire" many other "wires" may connect and influence further electrical activity. Thus, understanding brain circuitry may ultimately lead to improvements in treating Parkinson's disease. However, even our most complicated wiring diagrams are quite simple in scope when compared to the brain.

Let us now proceed to discuss research on Parkinson's disease.

THE CAUSE: WILL IT LEAD TO A CURE?

The first question often asked is, "What causes Parkinson's disease?" However, a more appropriate question would seem to be, "Is there a single cause of Parkinson's disease?" The answer to this is no. Any factor that damages the substantia nigra can lead to Parkinson's disease. At present there are at least three known causes of the disorder: *atherosclerotic, encephalitic,* and *idiopathic* (or unknown). The *encephalitic* variety is rare today, but was prevalent following a major outbreak of encephalitis in the 1920s. The *atherosclerotic* variety is associated with damage to many other areas of the brain and, thus, numerous other symptoms. The *idiopathic* cause is by far the major variety, but can now be broken down into the still unknown and the chemically caused. This is an area of considerable research.

A reversible type of Parkinsonism is caused by treatment with drugs that block the dopamine receptor. These drugs can be thought of as "false keys" since they fit into the lock but don't open the door; they prevent the right key from getting into the lock. Such drugs are used to treat brain diseases such as schizophrenia, but in the process of doing so, they produce Parkinson-like side effects. The treatment of Parkinsonism is simple: discontinue or lower the dose of the dopamine receptor-blocking drug, or administer drugs that block the actions of acetylcholine.

An irreversible type of Parkinson's disease appeared first in 1977 and now affects, or will affect, many people in California. In 1977, a twenty-three-year-old chemisty graduate student from the East Coast was referred to the National Institutes of Mental Health because he was mute, unable to move, and had a tremor. His symptoms were alleviated by levodopa. This graduate student had been making his own drugs in his basement and had been intravenously injecting them. He made a synthetic Demerol-like compound and got sloppy one time. He produced a by-product, which when injected caused Parkinson's disease. This young man continued to abuse several drugs, eventually died of a cocaine overdose in 1978. His brain looked like that of an elderly Parkinson's disease patient. This single case was published in a new journal and did not attract much attention.

As a "new heroin" appeared on the streets of California, several drug addicts came down with severe cases of Parkinson's disease. The symptoms in these patients also were caused by the same by-product, MPTP (short for N-methyl-4-phenyl-1,2,3,6-tetrahydropyridine). It became clear that a single injection of MPTP would not cause Parkinson's disease, but several injections would: as each dose did some damage to the brain's dopamine systems, many young addicts started to contract the disease. In the normal aging process, the brain loses dopamine cells in the substantia nigra. A loss of perhaps 80 percent of these cells is necessary to cause the symptoms of Parkinson's disease, so every individual living over 110–120 years would probably get the disease. However, in these young drug addicts, the brain had already lost many dopamine cells, so the process of normal aging would probably doom them to contract Parkinson's disease in the future. The loss of dopamine cells in the brains of some of these young people has been confirmed by a process called Positron Emission Tomography.

While all of these addicts injected MPTP intravenously, it would appear that other routes of exposure to the chemical also may result in Parkinson's disease. For example, a chemist who worked with MPTP many years ago rubbed his hands over the crystals to spread them out for drying and spent many years immobile in a mental institution. The chemical MPTP has proved valuable in producing an animal model of Parkinson's disease, but the real concern now is the role of such chemicals in the cause of Parkinson's disease in nondrug addicts.

In an excellent study conducted in Quebec, Canada,* there was a good correlation found between the incidence of Parkinson's disease and the use of herbicides and pesticides. In one farming region south of Montreal, the incidence of Parkinson's disease was about seven times higher than it was in neighboring regions with low herbicide/pesticide use. Along this line, it is important to note that it is not MPTP itself that causes Parkinson's disease, but a chemical substance called MPP+ produced in the body after MPTP is ingested. The MPP+ was field-tested as a herbicide under the trade name Cyperquat. The herbicide paraquat is structurally related to MPP+ and so are several other known chemicals. In a study of patients who got Parkinson's disease at or before the age of forty in Saskatchewan, 19 of 21 spent their first fifteen years in rural parts of the province, and all but one drank well water for the first fifteen years of their lives.

The incidence of Parkinson's disease is increasing. When the disease was first described by Dr. Parkinson, there were very few cases. Today the estimates are that one million or more persons have the disease in the United States alone. In part the numbers can be explained by the increase in life expectancy today as compared with the 1800s. There has been some recent evidence that the age of onset of Parkinson's disease is decreasing. This data are still difficult to interpret because early studies included numerous patients with postencephalitic disease in whom the age of onset was quite early. However, if the age of onset is decreasing, then some factor in the environment may be involved. Interestingly, the incidence of Parkinson's disease is not uniform throughout the world: the incidence in China is half that found in Europe and North America, while the incidence in Japan is even lower (35–45 percent).

---

*A. Barbeau and M. Roy, "Uneven Prevalence of Parkinson's Disease in the Province of Quebec," *Canadian Journal of Neurological Sciences* 12 (1985): 169–170.

Thus, there is mounting evidence that exposure to environmental contaminants, such as herbicides and pesticides, may be involved in the cause of Parkinson's disease. Since normal aging alone seems to predispose an individual to the disease, anything that decreases dopamine cells in the brain would tend to lower the age of onset of Parkinson's disease. Indeed, the cause of Parkinson's disease may be a series of factors that interrelate with each other.

GENETICS: IS PARKINSON'S DISEASE INHERITED?

A number of brain diseases are known to be inherited, but the overall picture seems to indicate that Parkinson's disease is not one of them. There are cases of identical twins where only one had the disease, and other cases where both did. Thus, genetics alone will not explain the incidence of the disease. However, this does not rule out a role for inheritance in the cause of Parkinson's disease. The problem in many such studies is that the disease becomes evident in later life and by that time it is difficult to determine all possible events that might have caused it. Even identical twins do not lead the same life after, or sometimes before, they leave home.

Along this line, it is interesting to note that in some studies there was one major difference between those twins who had contracted Parkinson's disease and those who had not. The twins without the disorder smoked more than the twins with the disease. This also had been confirmed in other studies where few Parkinson's disease patients smoked. It would appear that something in cigarette smoke may actually protect people from the disease. However, considering the risks of smoking, the "cure" may be worse than the disease. Further work along this line to determine the active ingredient might eventually prove useful.

A few research groups have reported that there is a relative deficit in liver enzymes in persons with Parkinson's disease. The liver is an important organ in preventing the toxicity of compounds. The liver contains chemicals called enzymes that change the structure of chemicals in the body. Some of these changes result in even more toxic chemicals, but the liver usually detoxifies such compounds very rapidly. One study noted that as the deficit in liver enzymes worsened, the onset of Parkinson's disease occurred earlier and earlier. Thus, a deficiency of liver enzymes may be involved in the disease. Since enzymes are genetically controlled—that is, inheritance determines the presence, absence, or activity level of various liver enzymes—

there is a potential role for genetics in the cause of Parkinson's disease. The inability to detoxify a chemical could be involved.

It would be unwise to rush from these few observations to the conclusion that the cause of Parkinson's disease is known, but it is known that the chemical MPTP can and will cause the disease. The effects of exposure to low levels of such chemicals over long periods of time are not known, but are certainly areas that require further study.

TREATMENT: BEYOND LEVODOPA

The first treatments of Parkinson's disease were found largely by trial and error, with the first successful treatment emerging in 1892, with the development of a drug that blocked acetylcholine receptors. This treatment was improved with new synthetic drugs in the 1940s, but was revolutionized by the discovery that levodopa would alleviate many of the symptoms. Despite the miracle of levodopa, problems remain with the treatment of Parkinson's disease. However, a review of current clinical treatments is not my aim here; a review of novel research areas is.

The basic structures of the substantia nigra, the striatum, and the nigrostriatal pathway, as well as those of much of the brain, have been explored in countless studies over the years. Many such studies have utilized the laboratory rat, largely because it is an economical model. The basic structures within the brain are quite similar from rats to humans, although the human brain areas involved in thinking are much more developed. Through research, the list of neurotransmitters has increased tremendously in the last twenty years, and especially during the last decade.

The study of dopamine systems in the brain was revolutionized in the early 1960s with the finding that dried brain sections exposed to formaldehyde gas changed dopamine into a chemical that glowed green under fluorescent light. This early technique and subsequent improvements have resulted in extensive maps of dopamine systems within the brains of numerous animals and humans. The role of such research in acquiring and developing an understanding of Parkinson's disease cannot be overstated. We know that dopamine acts on acetylcholine neurons. Thus, agents that block acetylcholine receptors improve (i.e., reduce) the symptoms of Parkinson's disease. However, the role of such drugs is secondary to that of levodopa.

Another area of interest is the role of other brain neurotransmitters, called neuropeptides, in influencing brain dopamine systems and, possibly, finding a secondary role in treating Parkinson's disease. A number of neuropeptides have been discovered in the brain. One of these, known as MIF (Melanocyte stimulating hormone release Inhibiting Factor) or PLG (L-Prolyl-L-Levoyl-Glycinamide), was shown to affect dopamine neurotransmission. In Parkinson's disease patients, MIF was described as dramatically improving the symptoms of the disease during concurrent levodopa treatment. These early studies involved intravenous MIF, which limited the usefulness of this agent. In numerous animal studies, it was shown that MIF affected dopamine neurotransmission, but the results have not been easy to interpret. In preliminary studies, we found that MIF increased the effect of dopamine neurotransmission, but the effects of MIF seemed to depend on the current state of the dopamine systems. Thus, these preliminary studies need to be followed up with more controlled studies, but MIF may yet play a role in treating Parkinson's disease. Certainly, MIF is not the only brain chemical that may prove useful in treating the disease, and much current, exciting research is in progress.

As mentioned above, it was not MPTP itself but a metabolite, MPP+, that caused Parkinson's disease. The chemical MPTP is processed in the body by an enzyme called monoamine oxidase, which exists in two forms and is found in the brain. There are drugs that bind to monoamine oxidase and prevent its actions. One of these, Deprenyl, prevents MPTP from poisoning brain cells. Much work is still needed to investigate the effects of Deprenyl in preventing the onset of or in effecting a treatment for Parkinson's disease. While a few studies have shown the dramatic effects of this drug on the disease, others have not.

DIAGNOSIS: LOOKING AT THE BRAIN

The clinical diagnosis of Parkinson's disease is well established, but the diagnosis of persons with preclinical cases of the disease is more difficult. The technique of Positron Emission Tomography (PET) scanning has provided valuable insights into this disease. However, it has not yet reached practical everday application because of the costs involved. In PET scanning, a very small dose of a radioactive drug is given to a patient, after which the location of the drug in the body is determined by using a series of detectors set up in a circle. With the help of a computer, the location of the drug can be relatively accurately determined.

In Parkinson's disease research, one could radiolabel levodopa or drugs that bind to dopamine receptors. With radiolabeled levodopa, it was shown in laboratory animals and humans exposed to MPTP that there was a substantial loss of dopamine in the substantia nigra prior to the onset of disease symptoms. Thus, there is good evidence that young drug addicts who use substances contaminated with MPTP will contract Parkinson's disease.

Positron Emission Tomography scanning is a potentially valuable research tool, but its practical significance is limited by the need for expensive equipment. The radioactivity involved in the procedure is safe, since it only lasts a few minutes to hours. Thus, patient safety is not the major concern. However, a cyclotron is needed to produce the radioactive drug, and a PET scanner must be used to locate affected areas of the brain. Both devices cost millions. In addition, the cyclotron must be close to the scanner, since the radioactivity does not last very long. Thus, such research will be limited to a few major research centers throughout the world.

ANIMAL MODELS OF PARKINSON'S DISEASE

One major research aim is to develop an animal model of each disease affecting humans. Such animal models are important to research because they allow the testing of drugs or procedures that are not yet allowed in humans. Without such models, the treatment of diseases such as Parkinson's would lag years behind current levels.

In terms of Parkinson's disease, rodent models were developed many years ago and have been widely studied. The primary rodent model (the rat or mouse) involved introducing a toxin called 6-hydroxydopamine into the brain to lesion (change or injure) the nigrostriatal pathway on one side. An animal with such a lesion will circle when placed into a circular chamber, or rotometer. Drugs that affect dopamine systems will affect the direction or magnitude of the circling. This was the best and most practical model of Parkinson's disease for many years, but it suffered from several limitations. For instance, the cardinal symptoms of the disease— the rigidity, the tremor, and the bradykinesia (slow movement) or akinesia (lack of movement), were not evident in the model. Thus, it was an accurate biochemical model but not an accurate behavioral model of the disease. Despite these limitations, numerous valuable studies were carried out using such models to increase our knowledge of Parkinson's disease. Despite advances in the development of other animal models, this rotational model will continue to be important.

The best current animal model of Parkinson's disease involves lesioning of the substantia nigra in the brain with intravenous MPTP. However, this model cannot be produced in the rat, probably because of differences in the rodent's ability to process the drug. In monkeys, MPTP produces the most accurate model of a human disease seen to date. Such models are being used in clinical trials of drugs and other potential treatments for Parkinson's disease. The accuracy of this model also would seem to implicate chemicals like MPTP in the cause of Parkinson's disease.

CONCLUSION

In summary, the cause of most cases of Parkinson's disease is not known, although much evidence has been uncovered. Parkinson's disease may not be caused by a single factor, except in cases of intravenous injection of MPTP. Normal aging may play a role, on top of which other factors increase the chance of getting the disease. Diet probably does not play a role other than possibly as a mechanism whereby toxic chemicals can enter the body. However, the cure may not be found just because the cause(s) are found. For instance, what causes the normal decrease in the numbers of dopamine neurons in the brain? Is it, as some speculate, dopamine itself or some other brain chemical? This certainly is an area of exciting research and may lead to some valuable clues. Whatever the cause of Parkinson's disease, the level of research for causes and treatments is exciting. The increase in our knowledge over the last few years has been tremendous, offering hope that a cure or, at least, better treatments may yet be found.

REFERENCES

Bloom, Floyd E. "Neopeptides." *Scientific American* 245 (1981): 148.
Langston, J. W.; P. Ballard; J. W. Tetrud; and I. Irwin. "Chronic Parkinsonism in Humans Due to a Product of Meperidine-analog Synthesis." *Science* 219 (1983): 979.
Levin, Roger. "Age Factors Loom in Parkinsonian Research." *Science* 234 (1986): 1200.
Ter-Pogossian, Michel M.; Marcus E. Raichle; and Burton E. Sobel. "Positron Emission Tomography." *Scientific American* 243 (1980): 170.

3

Neural Transplant in Parkinson's Disease

William C. Koller

The introduction of levodopa therapy in the early 1970s revolutionized the treatment of Parkinson's disease. This drug is very effective in decreasing the majority of Parkinsonian symptoms. However, optimal therapy for Parkinson's disease has yet to be achieved. Some symptoms of Parkinsonism, such as postural imbalance, mental changes, and involuntary nervous system dysfunction (i.e., constipation), do not respond well to levodopa treatment. After many years of levodopa therapy, treatment-related problems may develop. The hallucinations that may result from long-term therapy will require the dose of the levodopa to be lowered. Another major problem is that the disease symptoms are only controlled intermittently with long-term treatment, and the drug tends to lose its effectiveness in patients with advanced disease. While levodopa is a very good drug in the treatment of Parkinson's disease, it is not the ideal treatment. Therefore, doctors and researchers have been searching for better ways of treating Parkinsonism. New drugs have been developed as well as newer ways of delivering levodopa. Drugs that may prevent the progression of Parkinson's disease are now being evaluated. Another possible avenue of treatment is through a surgical intervention called neural transplantation.

ANIMAL STUDIES

Studies of neural transplantation have been performed on animals for some period of time. As far back as 1890, experiments were performed to place parts of cat brains into the brains of dogs. Many of the early investigations showed that it was possible to graft tissue, especially fetal tissue, from one animal to another. The grafts or tissue transfers could survive and grow in their new environment. The initial experiments of neural transplantation were performed to increase our understanding of how cells develop and mature. In 1945, a major step forward took place when it was demonstrated that neural grafting could be accomplished in a chamber of the eye. These experiments further supported the concept that grafts were capable of providing a form of nerve growth and that some elements in the tissue might promote such growth.

Investigations of neural transplantation in the 1970s attempted to focus on several key questions: (1) To what extent do grafted tissues survive after transplantation? (2) Do surviving cells have normal growth patterns? (3) Do the grafts grow and penetrate into brain tissue? (4) Can grafted cells change the functioning of the tissue in which they are transplanted? Attempts to answer these inquiries were aided by many advances in scientific methods and techniques. These studies illustrated the important discovery that neural connections could be reestablished by grafts of tissue from fetal nerve cells.

Many studies of neural transplantation have been directed to the brain area involved in Parkinson's disease, most particularly the chemical dopamine released by the striatum. We don't know why the nerve cells in the substantia nigra die, but when they do it results in a loss of dopamine in the striatum. The loss of dopamine causes nerve dysfunction and the symptoms of Parkinson's disease result. Initial studies of animal models of Parkinsonism showed that neural grafts can change normal behavior, presumably because the grafted cells survive and produce dopamine. Other experiments have shown that grafted nerve tissue will grow and enhance nerve growth in other parts of the brain.

The discovery that the chemical MPTP would produce in both humans and animals all the behavioral, anatomical (degeneration of the substantia nigra), and neurochemical (loss of dopamine in the striatum) aspects of Parkinsonism was a major research advance. For the first time an exact animal model of Parkinson's disease existed. MPTP-treated monkeys provided an opportunity for testing the effect of fetal nerve cell grafts. Redmond and co-workers have shown in this animal model that fetal substantia nigra grafts will reverse the Parkinsonian signs and cause an increase in striatal dopamine. These grafts appear to survive and grow without any problems associated with tissue rejection. The investigators felt that grafting fetal tissue may have considerable merit for clinical application in Parkinson's disease. But they also suggested that numerous scientific questions should be addressed before human trials could be undertaken. A few of the issues that need to be resolved include: What tissue should be transplanted (e.g., fetal versus adrenal)? How should the graft tissue be prepared? How much tissue should be transferred? What is the best site for grafting? Should drugs be given to suppress tissue rejection? Will Parkinson's disease affect the graft? It is hoped that investigations with animals will provide the answers to these and other questions.

HUMAN STUDIES

Neural transplants have been performed in humans despite the relative lack of scientific information. The first clinical tests of neural transplants were performed in Sweden in 1985. Borklund and his co-workers placed tissue from a patient's own adrenal medulla gland into the substance of the striatum. The adrenal gland sits on top the kidney in the abdomen. This gland secretes many chemicals including dopamine. The middle part of the adrenal gland, the medulla, is a source of dopamine-producing cells and is thus a candidate for grafting. Abdominal surgery is necessary in order to remove the adrenal gland. Two patients operated on in Sweden were a fifty-five-year-old man with an eight-year history of the disease, and a forty-six-year-old woman with a five-year history of symptoms. Both patients were said to have severe disease. In neither case was any significant improvement in Parkinsonian signs noted. One patient showed freer movement of both arms beginning two days after surgery. Tremor and hypokinesia were absent until the fourth postoperative day, when symptoms returned and levodopa was reinstituted in increasing doses. Two weeks after surgery, the other patient suffered from periods of paranoia, and the slowing of movements appeared to be more pronounced. Over the next two weeks, the patient returned to her preoperative state and levodopa therapy was reinstituted. In general, the results in these patients were disappointing.

In marked contrast to the results of the Swedish workers, Dr. Madrazo in Mexico City reported in a 1987 issue of the prestigious *New England Journal of Medicine* the highly successful treatment of two patients. Using a somewhat different technique, he put the adrenal tissue into the side of the striatum (rather than into the middle) where the graft was in contact with the brain (ventricular) fluid. The patients were young (thirty-five and thirty-nine, respectively) and were said to have severe disease. Clinical improvement was noted at six and fifteen days respectively and was said to continue with time. Rigidity and bradykinesia were reported to have virtually disappeared and tremor was greatly reduced. Therefore, a marked improvement was noted and patients no longer needed medications. Reduction of Parkinsonian symptoms occurred on both sides of the body rather than just on the side of the body opposite to the implant as might have been expected. No complications of the surgery were reported. The study did not use standard methods to assess Parkinsonian symptoms, but the results were so spectacular that perhaps this was not necessary. There was, however, no neurologist or expert in Parkinson's disease associated with the Mexican team. The report initiated a tremendous reaction from doctors interested in Parkinson's disease. Some thought that this procedure represented a major advancement in treatment; others expressed cautious optimism, while still others decried the procedure as having no proven value. However, because of the marked improvement reported, neurologists and neurosurgeons teamed together in the United States in order to perform and assess the adrenal transplant procedure.

In the fall of 1987, doctors who had begun to perform the transplant surgery met in Chicago to discuss the safety and efficacy of the procedure. This was an open meeting in which matters relevant to the transplant treatment were discussed. This format provided quick access to all available information and an honest appraisal of the procedure. There was some controversy but all agreed on the need for more information. Several groups decided to proceed with the surgery. By 1988, the Mexican group had operated on forty-four patients and continued to report marked improvement. Functional ability was said to increase and individuals were said to have returned to work. Improvement was reported to have continued after the operation. Complications were not commented upon, but it was learned that four of the forty-four patients (10 per cent) had died and other serious adverse reactions had also occurred. It became evident that some of these patients had been made worse by the surgery. Data from the American studies became available in late 1987 and early 1988. For the most part some improvement in Parkinsonian signs occurred: particularly there was less time spent in the "off" state, and when it did occur, the state tended to be less severe. Patients still needed medications, however, and the improvement was not as marked as had been reported by the Mexican doctors. Yet, in general, the researchers were somewhat encouraged. On the other hand, it became apparent that serious complications could occur with the operation: several deaths were reported and some patients had strokes associated with the procedure. The postoperative course in almost all patients was exceedingly complicated. Pneumonia was commonplace, as were many gastrointestinal problems. Patients often spent several months in the hospital. As a result of these findings, several teams stopped performing the operation.

The value of neurotransplantation remains uncertain. A *New York Times* editorial entitled "New Parkinson Technique: Enthusiasm Turns to Disillusion" led to discouragement with the procedure. One thing was clear, Americans could not reproduce results of the Mexicans even when the same procedure was used. The reason for this discrepancy is unclear. Lack of adequate scientific methods or possibly investigator bias may have played a part. The risk of the operation, especially for older individuals, became apparent. Nonetheless, some patients did improve with the operation. Combined data from Kansas City, Chicago, and Tampa research groups indicated that six months after surgery there was a significant decrease in the "off" time—its severity decreased. These neurologists reported no change in function during the "on" or good period and there was no change in the dosage of anti-Parkinsonian medications.

The status of adrenal transplant in Parkinson's disease is therefore not totally determined. It would appear, however, that this procedure has only limited applicability for treatment of the Parkinsonian population in general, and that the procedure is still highly investigative. The risk of the procedure to the patient should be clearly understood by anyone considering the operation. It should also be pointed out that for some patients any benefit derived may be transient at best, lasting only several months. Considering the risk and postoperative complications, the procedure could not be deemed worthwhile if only several months of benefit resulted.

Neural transplantation in animals has shown favorable results using fetal tissue, especially when applied to the substantia nigra. Several fetal transplants have been performed on humans. The Mexican group again reported excellent results in two patients, one receiving fetal substantia nigra and the other fetal adrenal medullary tissue. Fetal transplants have also been performed in England and Sweden. The use of fetal tissue grafts has not been thoroughly studied; however, at this writing, several patients in the United States (Colorado) and Sweden have received fetal grafts. Numerous legal, ethical, and religious concerns must be addressed. The laws of most states do allow use of spontaneously aborted fetal tissue. However, the idea that conception of an embryo might be sought as a means for providing donor tissue, or that some material gain might be achieved, represent possible problems. Several alternatives to the use of human fetal tissue may exist, such as cells from laboratory cultures. Only time and more investigation will delineate the true value, if any, of the neural transplantation procedures in Parkinson's disease. It is certainly possible that new means of performing neural transplantation may be developed that will offer better results.

REFERENCES

Borklund, E. D.; Granberg, P. O.; and Hamberger, B. "Transplantation of Adrenal Medullary Tissue to Striatum in Parkinsonism." *Journal of Neurosurgery* 62 (1985): 169–173.

Freed, W. J. "Adrenal Grafts in Animals." *Science* 221 (1988): 241.

Madrazo, I.; Drucker-Colin, A.; and Diaz, V. "Open Mircosurgical Autograft of Adrenal Medulla to Right Caudate Nucleus in Two Patients with Intractable Parkinson's Disease." *The New England Journal of Medicine* 316 (1987): 831–834.

Redmond, D. E.; Sladek, J. R.; and Roth, R. A. "Transplanted Cells: A Future Treatment for Parkinson's Disease." *Neurological Consultant* 4 (1987): 1-8.

4

Nursing Care

Nelda D. Dippel

The management of Parkinson's disease is a challenge not only to those afflicted but to the family and to the health care professionals involved in their care. Although highly effective drugs exist to relieve the symptoms, the length and quality of the Parkinsonian patient's life depends on the maintenance of optimal general health.

The patient and family members typically have the primary responsibility of managing the day to day problems that emerge as Parkinsonism progresses. Unfortunately, these persons may not have all the information needed to tackle new challenges. In this chapter I intend to provide practical information for the care of the Parkinsonian patient and to illustrate, however briefly, ways in which the professional nurse can serve patients and their families.

MEDICATION

Parkinsonian patients and their families (or caregivers) should be aware of several potential side effects of levodopa preparations. Nausea, for example, is a common reaction to the medication, especially early in the treatment process. Taking care to administer the medication after a meal low in protein or with a snack will reduce this problem. However, if nausea and vomiting persist, the physician should be notified since a dangerous (electrolyte) imbalance of chemicals, such as sodium and potassium can occur within the body. The physician may choose to reduce the medication or to order special drugs designed to stop the nausea.

Parkinsonian patients undergoing drug therapy may notice a drop in blood pressure when rapid changes of position are attempted (e.g., standing up from a sitting position). This is called orthostatic hypotension. Such movement should be undertaken slowly. For example, patients should sit on the side of the bed a minute before standing, then stand still a minute before starting to walk; both of these precautions will reduce dizziness. If dizziness occurs, sit down to reduce the chance of falling. Elastic stockings squeeze the legs and prevent pooling of blood, thereby reducing the severity of these symptoms. If a blood pressure cuff is available, the patient's blood pressure can be monitored and significant changes reported to the registered nurse or physician. These symptoms may or may not occur, and when present they often disappear after several days or weeks.

During the course of the disease, involuntary movements (dyskinesias) occur in many individuals undergoing levodopa therapy; they are related to the duration of the therapy rather than the dosage. The tongue, the face, the mouth, or the entire body may be affected. Dyskinesias are slow, rhythmic, automatic, stereotyped movements. Facial grimacing, exaggerated chewing, protrusion of the tongue, rhythmic opening and closing of the mouth, jerky arm and leg movements, and exaggerated respiration are examples of possible dyskinesias. The only way to stop these symptoms is to reduce the dosage of levodopa, but this would reduce the effectiveness of the treatment and the symptoms of Parkinson's disease would recur. Most individuals prefer to tolerate the medication's side effects rather than be disabled by the disease.

Irregular heart beats, agitation, confusion, and insomnia are occasional side effects of the medication. These symptoms should always be reported to the physician. In addition, caregivers should be on the lookout for black tarry stools, which often indicate bleeding from the gastrointestinal tract. Rapid blinking of the eyes (blepharospasm) can be an early sign of an overdose of levodopa and should be reported. Some individuals notice darkening of the urine, saliva, and perspiration due to increases in levodopa metabolism.

Little improvement is expected to occur during the first few days of medication therapy, but the patient may continue to improve up to six months after the medication is started. It is important to know the name, the dosage, and the most common side effects of prescribed medications. The physician should be aware of any over-the-counter drugs patients are using, since undesirable interactions could result when certain medications are combined. Patients and/or caregivers should take all medications to the physician on the initial visit, including vitamins and over-the-counter drugs.

Mood changes and confusion related to the disease could contribute to medication errors. Family members should always administer the drugs if there is any question of the patient's reliability in this regard. A simple system can be developed to assist the affected individual and at the same time allow more independence. A separate envelope with the correct medication for breakfast, lunch, dinner, and bedtime doses can be prepared and labeled appropriately to assist the mildly confused or forgetful individual.

Illness, surgery, hospitalization, or other emotional upsets may make it necessary for the physician to discontinue medication for a few days. If this occurs, increased symptoms may occur until the patient can readjust to the medication.

NUTRITION

Parkinsonian symptoms and medication side effects may require changes in such everyday practices as food selection and preparation. The individual with Parkinson's disease needs a well-balanced daily diet containing protein for strength, fiber to prevent or control constipation, and approximately three quarts of liquids.

Although it is important to have sufficient quantities of protein daily, high protein meals have been shown to block the effect of levodopa. The amount of protein in the total diet may need to be decreased or redistributed. This reduction in protein will depend on the particular prescribed dosage of medication. A protein redistribution diet is not necessary for all patients, therefore the physician should be consulted before any dietary changes are made. If the physician advises protein reduction or redistribution, the foods that should be limited include milk, red meat, fish, poultry, cheese, eggs, peanuts, nuts, sunflower seeds, whole grains, and soybean products.

If constipation is a problem, prune juice should be included in the daily diet, since it is a natural laxative. The amount of dietary fiber should also be increased to include one bowl of bran flakes, leafy vegetables, and one serving of fruit or fruit salad ever day. Bran muffins or bran combined in meatloaves may provide extra fiber and a tasty treat.

Delores Alford, President of the Institution of Gerontic Nursing, states that the following recipe may assist the older individual who suffers from constipation:

1/2 lb. raisins
1/2 lb. prunes
1/2 lb. figs
1/2 cup dates
1 oz. senna leaves

Grind together and stir several times. Roll into one inch balls. Eat one or more daily as needed. May be frozen for later use.

Weight loss may occur in persons with Parkinson's disease. It is well known that the appetite is altered by neurotransmitter levels. Problems with swallowing, tremor, and bradykinesia may also result in the patient reducing food intake as eating becomes more difficult. Severe tremors require increased caloric intake to maintain weight. If it becomes a problem, calorie intake may need to be raised. Sustacal (a food supplement), milkshakes, and eggnog may assist in maintaining or increasing weight. Although it is rather unusual for those with Parkinson's to be overweight, it can occur because physical activity is limited. If the person is overweight, calories should be reduced since regulation of medication will be more difficult. Weight loss will facilitate movement and reduce the risk of heart disease. Reduction of salt intake will also reduce the workload on the heart.

Vitamins or dietary supplements should not be taken unless prescribed by a physician. Large doses of vitamin preparations containing B_6 can diminish levodopa's ability to reach the brain. Avocados, lentils, and lima beans are high in vitamin B_6 and should be limited for this reason. This limitation is not necessary when taking the Sinemet or Madopar variations of levodopa.

At least three quarts of liquids per day are needed to maintain proper body functions. The liquids can include water, fruit juice, or (decaffeinated or regular) coffee. Alcoholic beverages should be limited. No more than two cocktails or glasses of wine should be consumed per day. Drinking during the day or when alone should be discouraged since alcohol may neutralize the effects of the levodopa.

Tremors and an impaired ability to swallow can at times make eating difficult. Caregivers may relieve eating problems by modifying food preparation and service. Semi-solid foods such as baked or mashed potatoes, cooked fruits, bananas, puddings, and meatloaves may be easier to eat.

Meat should be cut into small pieces and chewed thoroughly before swallowing. Some individuals find that it is less tiring if they eat smaller meals four times a day, instead of the usual three meals.

To prevent choking on food particles, and to promote comfort, oral hygiene should be planned immediately following meals. If swallowing causes difficulty in taking medication, crush the pill and serve it in a small amount of applesauce or pudding. The only exception here is the drug Sinemet CR, which should not be crushed; to do so destroys the controlled release properties and could result in dyskinesias or other side effects. Another suggestion is to have the patient drink something (like juice) before taking pills. The fluid lightly coats the throat in preparation for the medication. Afterward some banana could be eaten to assure that the pill is thoroughly ingested. For those who experience a dry mouth, chewing gum or sucking on hard candies might help: the symptom usually cannot be avoided but it does not threaten health.

There should be ample time allocated for meals so that the Parkinsonian patient does not feel hurried. When slowness of movement and tremor are present, the use of warming trays may prevent food from becoming cold and unappetizing. Dishes with weighted bottoms, usually beneficial, are available from stores that sell medical supplies. Large napkins are useful, but do not attempt to apply them in a bib-like style unless specifically requested by the patient. To do so could cause considerable embarrassment. Remember at all times that the patient is an adult who deserves respect and whose self-esteem is vital to the treatment process.

As an aside, denture wearers should take care to ensure that dentures are properly fitted. Weight loss may change the shape of the gums, thus requiring dentures to be realigned. Consult with a dentist before removing dentures, since dental plates that are left out of the mouth for three days or more may no longer fit because of tissue changes in the mouth.

ELIMINATION

Constipation is a common complaint of those with Parkinson's disease: a diminished ability of intestinal muscles to move feces is often combined with side effects of many medications used to treat the disease. Enemas should be discouraged in favor of modifications in diet and lifestyle to best ensure normal elimination. As previoiusly discussed, increased levels of fiber and liquids are important to reduce constipation.

Walking should be encouraged since this helps propel the stool and strengthens the abdominal and pelvic muscles needed in the act of defecation. If the patient is unable to walk, then isometric excercises designed to tighten and relax the muscles of the stomach and buttocks may help.

A specific time each day should be set for bowel elimination. It is usually better to set this time after breakfast or immediately following a warm drink, in order to stimulate the bowels to move. Leaning forward or sitting with feet on a low footstool will increase abdominal pressure and assist in the elimination process. Straining should be avoided to prevent hemorroids. Assistive devices such as arm rails located near the toilet provide helpful leverage. Those who have trouble changing from a sitting to a standing position may benefit from a raised toilet seat, which can be purchased from any medical supply store.

It is easier to prevent constipation than to treat it. Long-term use of laxatives can lead to a loss of muscle tone or an irritated bowel and thus cause diarrhea. Mineral oil preparations should not be used as laxatives, because they can be dangerous if the individual has trouble swallowing: if any of these fluids are sucked into the lungs, pneumonia could result. If a laxative must be used, select a mild one such as milk of magnesia, citrate of magnesium, or glycerine suppositories. Stool softeners—e.g., Surfax and Colace—can be used several times a day since they are safe drugs and can be used indefinitely.

A fecal impaction should be suspected if a bowel movement has not occurred in three days. Sometimes, if a person is partially impacted, only the liquid can pass through, creating the impression that diarrhea is present. If there are no results from a soap suds or oil retention enema, it may be necessary to break up the impaction manually by inserting a gloved finger gently into the rectum. Do not try to remove an impaction without consulting with the physician, since this activity can be dangerous in certain conditions.

Urinary Problems

Urinary problems may occur in severe cases of Parkinson's disease. The enlarged prostate in the older male may complicate the situation. Difficulty starting the stream, increased frequency, inability to control urination, and incontinence may be present. Decreased physical activity and poor bladder muscle tone may make these individuals more susceptible to urinary tract infections. A physician should be notified if burning occurs with urination, if the patient is unable to urinate or if urination is too frequent, if the patient is experiencing the feeling that urination cannot wait, or if pain is present.

If clothing is commonly soiled with urine, a condom catheter or a sanitary pad can be worn to provide protection and odor control. A urinal or commode at bedside is useful for preventing accidents. Include two or three glasses of cranberry juice (or any substance high in vitamin C [ascorbic acid]) in the daily diet if urinary infections occur.

DROOLING

If drooling is a problem, the fear of choking may present itself. When in bed, those who are bothered with drooling should be on their side to decrease the pooling of saliva in the back of the mouth. A bulb syringe can be used to remove the pooled saliva, so aspiration of these secretions can be avoided. Family members may feel more secure if they receive training in first aid and the Heimlich Maneuver. Classes on these subjects are available from the American Red Cross or American Heart Association.

HEAT TOLERANCE

Those with Parkinson's disease may be hypersensitive to heat and develop a fever in hot weather. Report this to the nurse or the physician to rule out other causes of an elevated temperature. Warm baths and massage may relax muscles and relieve those who suffer from excess perspiration. Do not use alcohol for massage, because it can be too drying for sensitive elderly skin.

VISION

If blurred vision or other symptoms related to the eyes occur, a physician may refer the patient to an ophthalmologist for an examination, which will include testing for glaucoma, dryness, and visual changes. If reduced blinking is a problem, artificial tears can be used to prevent corneal drying. Be sure to discuss the problem with a physician. Take precautions to prevent eye infection: wash hands well before using any type of eye medication or artificial tears, and use moistened cotton swabs to remove any greasy scales from external eyelid margins.

SEBORRHEA

If seborrhea (an increase in the oily secretions of the skin) is present, use frequent baths, drying soaps, and antidandruff shampoos.

SLEEP DISTURBANCE

Parkinsonian patients frequently complain of sleep disturbance (see chapter 8). Try to avoid too many periods of sleep during the day; this should assure better sleep habits at night.

SEXUAL PROBLEMS

Sexual problems are sometimes present as a result of the effects of chronic disease, depression, or the fear of being unable to satisfy one's sexual partner. Occasionally side effects of medications may be involved. If problems surface, a discussion with a physician may lead to helpful suggestions concerning more appropriate techniques, assistive measures, or therapy to enhance sexual enjoyment.

DEPRESSION

Depression can be a part of the disease process or a side effect of medications (see chapter 10). The physician should always be notified when depression is present. If there is discussion of suicidal thoughts, the physician should be consulted immediately.

SPEECH

Some Parkinsonian patients complain of speech problems (see chapter 5). Speech may be barely audible, monotonous, and rapid. Breathing exercises to improve breath control, along with tongue, jaw, and lip exercises may be beneficial. Such exercises may prove helpful, but they can also be tiring, and for that reason they should not be practiced too long. Discontinue exercise when pain or extreme fatigue occurs.

Muscle weakness and rigidity may cause those with Parkinson's disease to sit with their mouths open. To relax the muscle of the jaw and throat, so that air passages will be open for breathing and speaking, have the patient recite words such as: *open, over, clover, free, evening, beam.* These words should be recited approximately five times per day. Practice saying "oo" and "ee" with exaggerated lip movements. Taking deep breaths before speaking should increase speech volume. Other activities that may be beneficial include reading aloud, singing in the shower, making faces in the mirror, and reciting the alphabet. Some patients have found it helpful to use a tape recorder: by playing back the tape, areas needing improvement can be recognized and improved.

Breathing exercises are recommended, such as raising the arms straight above the shoulders while air is inhaled through the nose, then lowering the arms while exhaling the air through the mouth in a hissing manner.

An electronic amplifier of the type employed by individuals who have their larynx removed may be used if speech is too low to be understood. An appointment should be made with a speech therapist if problems are serious: Available communication devices can be discussed and specific exercises suggested to overcome special problem areas. Improvement may be slow and inconsistent, but most individuals can be helped so that their speech can be better understood. The improved speech will facilitate socialization and enhance mental outlook.

BALANCE

People with Parkinson's disease have a displaced center of gravity and postural instability, thus falls can occur (see chapter 7). Approximately 25 percent of those with the disease may experience these problems, and 15 percent may experience serious injuries from falls. It is very important therefore that the living environment be evaluated to remove potential dangers. Turning, backing up, and getting out of chairs are the most common occasions for falls. The following tips may prove beneficial to Parkinsonian patients:

1. Sit down if feeling faint.

2. Either remove scatter rugs or tack them down securely.

3. Add lamps to areas that are not properly lighted.

4. For those who experience unsteadiness, a whistle should be worn around the neck to summon help in the event of a fall.

5. Exercise should be undertaken only when supervised.

6. Install grab bars around the tub, the bed, and the commode. Do not use towel racks for support since they are not properly anchored.

7. Use nonskid bathtub surfaces.

8. If the patient is unsteady, place a stool in the tub. Use of a hand-held shower nozzle will allow proper bathing while seated on a stool.

9. Replace glass shower doors with plastic doors or curtains.

10. Sit while dressing or grooming. Long-handled combs and razors may be useful.

11. Sturdy chairs placed in the kitchen, the bedroom, and in television viewing areas will help to maintain independence.

IMPAIRED MOBILITY

Perhaps the most disturbing feature of Parkinson's disease is the difficulty patients experience when attempting to move. Daily exercise will maintain joint mobility and reduce uncomfortable tightness (see chapter 6). Range of motion exercises, which move the joints in directions of normal rotation, need to be accomplished twice a day. It may be necessary for family members to move the patient through the motions in more severe cases. Walking, riding a stationary bicycle, swimming, or gardening are all beneficial but should not be overdone. Frequent rest periods should be taken.

It is important that the Parkinsonian patient complete as many daily activities as possible. Slow movement of the fingers may make dressing difficult, but the individual needs to be encouraged to do everything possible to maintain independence. Even the act of dressing provides some exercise. Loose clothing with elastic waistbands that open in the front may facilitate dressing. Use of velcro fasteners, zippers, snaps instead of buttons, and slip-on shoes without laces will help as well. Long-handled shoe horns are available if needed.

An occupational therapist may provide other suggestions that will assist in maintaining independence in activities of daily living. Since patients' ability to move will fluctuate widely, they may be able to do some tasks on certain days that cannot be done on others. It will be important to arrange daily schedules to allow sufficient time for completion of self-care routines.

A registered nurse or physical therapist can teach both patients and caregivers exercises that can be done at home. It is important to remember that it takes courage to walk and exercise after experiencing falls, but inactivity will cause the muscles to grow weak.

Those with Parkinson's disease should be instructed to walk erect with their feet about ten inches apart and with eyes focused on the horizon. Arms should be swung while walking, and heels should be lifted, as if marching. It is better to place the heel down first and to walk with fairly long strides. If there is difficulty in starting to walk, try rocking back and forth before stepping off. Practice walking into tight corners helps to overcome fear of close places. The hands may be exercised by tearing paper or jingling coins.

A trapeze bar installed over the bed or a strong rope tied to the foot of the bed, with a knot in the end, will allow independence in sitting up. Special chairs with catapult spring seats, available at most medical supply houses, are helpful for those who have difficulty standing up from a normal chair. To assist standing from a seated position, the feet should be wide apart and the individual should push against the arms of the chair. Rise with speed to overcome the pull of gravity.

Warm baths and massage will relax muscles and increase comfort. Stretching exercises designed to loosen the joint structures should follow baths and will help to prevent contracted limbs. Use of elastic stockings and elevating the feet may help reduce the swelling of the lower extremities that occurs at the end of the day. Persistent swelling should be evaluated by the physician to determine the cause.

Bedridden patients should be moved frequently to prevent skin breakdown and muscle atrophy. The skin should be observed for redness in areas of pressure, such as the buttocks, elbows, and heels. Air mattresses may be useful to relieve pressure at these sensitive areas. The bedridden person should be encouraged to breathe deeply and to cough every two hours to reduce the likelihood of fluid building up in the lungs thus preventing the onset of pneumonia.

NURSING MANAGEMENT

If specialized nursing care is required at some stage of the disease, local visiting nurse services may provide invaluable assistance. These services are available in most communities and will require a physician's order. Such services may be paid by medicare or other insurance and permit continued treatment at home rather than in the hospital.

Nursing management will include careful assessment of needs, assistance with drug therapy, patient and family education, and exercises to loosen joint structures. A bowel routine, warm baths and massages, assistance in obtaining self-help devices, and making appropriate referrals are all part of the nursing management of the Parkinsonian client. Emotional support, provided by caring nurses, can be especially important in encouraging adherence to treatment regimes.

SUGESTED READING

Fischbach, F. T. "Easing Adjustment of Parkinson's Disease." *American Journal of Nursing,* 76 (1978): 66–69.

Gresh, C. "Helpful Hints You Can Give Your Patients with Parkinson's Disease." *Nursing 80,* 10, no. 1 (1980): 26–33.

Hahn, K. "Protocol: Management of Parkinson's Disease." *Nurse Practitioner,* 7, nos. 1–6 (1982): 13–20.

Ho, R. "Physical Therapy." In *Parkinson's Disease Handbook.* New York: American Parkinson Disease Association, 1980, p. 28.

Langan, R. J. "Parkinson's Disease: Assessment, Procedure and Guidelines for Counseling." *Nurse Practitioner,* 2 (1976): 13–16.

Langan, R. J.; and Cotzias, G. C. "Do's and Dont's for the Patient on Levodopa Therapy." *American Journal of Nursing,* 76, no. 6 (1976): 917–918.

5

Speech and Communication

Kathryn L. Blakesley

Approximately 50 percent of all persons with Parkinson's disease develop difficulty with speech. There are several types of speech problems that Parkinsonians commonly confront. (Not all patients exhibit every symptom.) With some patients, the symptoms are subtle, while in others they may be severely debilitating. For most, the onset of symptoms is gradual with a slow but steady progression.

Parkinsonian patients often cannot speak loudly enough to be heard. They may have trouble talking over normal television or radio volume and may experience great difficulty talking when in a group. This is commonly the first reported speech change. Initially, such patients may experience a fading voice: it is strong at the beginning of the utterance but becomes weaker, or in some cases inaudible, the longer one speaks. Imprecise pronunciation is a frequent complaint, as well as decreased volume. Unclear speech sounds make it difficult for others to understand what is said. Words may be slurred and the final sound in words is often dropped. There are often short rushes of very rapid speech, and inappropriate silences, thus syllables and words are frequently crowded and run together. The loss of natural pauses between syllables and words, coupled with poor pronunciation, may render the Parkinsonians' speech undiscernible at times. Changes in voice quality may also be exhibited: the voice may sound breathy, tremulous, or higher in pitch. Hoarseness is not uncommon.

Likewise, Parkinsonians may have difficulty initiating speech. There are often unwanted hesitations before speaking; at other times uncontrollable repetitions occur. Words, phrases, or even whole sentences may be repeated unintentionally. Their speech is affected in much the same way as the more obviously manifested symptoms (e.g., tremor and bradykinesia). A quivering, tremulous voice quality and slow speech rate are comparable to the abnormal shaking, stiff muscles, and slow-moving limbs characteristic of Parkinson's disease. Similarly, difficulty initiating speech is comparable to the stumbling or frozen gait that is common in Parkinsonism. The patients' stooped posture may cause problems with inhalation, the very power source governing voice volume.

Lack of volume control, unnatural breaks in speech, and lack of inflection make it difficult for Parkinsonian patients to communicate at times. Involuntary pauses in speech make being understood extremely difficult and a source of considerable embarrassment for those afflicted with the disease. As communication becomes more difficult some Parkinsonians retreat to a world of almost total silence.

FACIAL EXPRESSIONS

Characteristically, a progressive loss of facial expression occurs with Parkinsonism. The patient's face often appears masklike and expressionless. Smiling, frowning, grinning, and the ability to express anger, fear, and joy require conscious effort and muscle coordination. While these gestures do not directly affect speech, changes in facial expression are important forms of body language: they help to get ideas across, enhance the ability to communicate, and help the listener attach meaning and intent to what is being said. As the ability to maintain facial expression declines, the communication sequence is interrupted in yet another way: the listener may become confused and unable to respond appropriately, resulting in the eventual breakdown of social interaction with those who suffer from Parkinson's.

SWALLOWING

Reduced movement of the throat muscles can occur in Parkinsonian patients, and the result may be difficulty with swallowing. Patients may experience problems chewing or manipulating food in the mouth, which is associated with eating difficulties and an accumulation of saliva.

A well-known expert in swallowing disorders, Jerilyn Logemann, states that Parkinsonian patients exhibit a typical repetitive rolling pattern during swallowing. Food, or saliva, is held in a normal position when the swallow is begun. The tongue then rolls the food toward the back of the mouth; however, the back of the tongue often does not lower and the food rolls forward again. The back and forth movement may be repeated a number of times until the stages of the swallow can continue. It is thought that this may indicate a form of muscle rigidity that prevents the tongue from being lowered once it has been elevated. Dr. Logemann further states in her book *Evaluation and Treatment of Swallowing Disorders* that in general there is a progression of swallowing dysfunction. As the disease progresses, a patient's larynx may not close during swallowing, which allows some material to enter the airway during the swallow or material may fall into the open airway when the patient inhales after the swallow.

Difficulty with swallowing is often compounded by the build-up of saliva in the mouth. Normally, saliva is swallowed automatically, but due to their slow rate of swallowing, Parkinsonians pool saliva in the mouth and throat. If the excess saliva is allowed to accumulate, it can spill forward between the lips, resulting in drooling. As embarrassing and frustrating as it may be for Parkinsonians to have food or saliva dribble from their mouths, the collection of saliva can also significantly undermine intelligible speech. The patients must remember to swallow any excess saliva before speaking; make a conscious effort to swallow saliva often by closing the lips firmly and propelling the saliva to the back of the throat; and maintain their heads in an upright position so saliva will collect in the back of the throat thereby facilitating automatic swallowing. These measures are difficult, monotonous, and exhausting but all are necessary for those who are afflicted with Parkinson's disease.

EVALUATION AND TREATMENT

It is obvious that patients do better and can face their problems more effectively when they gain a reasonable understanding of their affliction. Consequently, the success of any treatment depends more than ever on the cooperation of patients and families. It is advisable that, in addition to medical intervention, Parkinsonians be evaluated by a team of professionals who can make appropriate recommendations for comprehensive treatment. In conjunction with medication, valuable positive reinforcement can be gained by having the patients participate in exercise therapy, speech therapy, recreational therapy, and psychological counseling. These therapies not only help modify habits but provide mediums that encourage social interaction. Many areas of the country now have local organizations that help serve both Parkinsonians and their families, providing multidisciplinary treatment programs and helpful information. Parkinson's disease is a shared burden and must be addressed on many levels. ʼ

A speech pathologist, often referred to as a speech therapist, is one member of the team of professionals who can help Parkinsonians. Speech pathologists work in a number of settings. They are employed by the public schools, hospitals, agencies, and clinics; some are in private practice. Patients or their families should seek a state licensed, qualified therapist who is certified by the American Speech-Language and Hearing Association and is experienced with voice disorders and Parkinson's disease.

Once a qualified therapist has been found, an initial evaluation should be conducted to determine the areas most in need of assistance. The evaluation should be followed by recommendations and treatment specific to individual needs. There is no one pattern of speech disturbance in Parkinson's disease; however, it is necessary for a qualified therapist to assess the patient's present level of functioning and adapt appropriate exercises and equipment to the patients' needs and interests at successive stages of the disease. It is generally felt that if therapy is started early, at the point where speech is just beginning to break down, impairment can be delayed and both patients and their families can understand and adjust as the disease progresses.

Whenever possible it is beneficial for patients to participate in group therapy sessions. Group therapy provides an opportunity for socialization. The group situation provides comradery; in fact, many patients report losing feelings of isolation while enjoying the friendship and social acceptance of others in the group. Group training can also provide an opportunity for Parkinsonian patients to gain encouragement, stamina, and motivation through peer support. It is easier for patients to make an effort when they see others trying, overcoming their fears and failures, and then succeeding after a second or third attempt. Motivation is increased when fellow patients say, "You can do it," "Try it again," or "You're among friends."

The group approach also provides an atmosphere in which awareness of certain speech habits, pitfalls, and tried and true suggestions for dealing with speech and swallowing difficulties can be discussed. Comments such as "I know exactly what you mean," and "Do you have that problem too?" give comfort and spur patients on to continue with therapy, to practice at home, and to accept the problems they must face. The group is an accepting environment where feelings can be vented and grievances aired.

The group approach is not without its disadvantages. Withdrawn persons may find it hard to express themselves as members of a group. Others may be overwhelmed by group pressure, or become easily provoked in this type of setting. Despite the possible shortcomings, it is generally felt that working in groups is favorable. At any rate, the speech therapist can determine the most advantageous course of treatment for an individual following his assessment. It is possible that a combination of individual and group therapy may be indicated.

SPECIAL CIRCUMSTANCES AND RECOMMENDATIONS

Voice

For patients in the advanced stages of Parkinson's disease or who have a weak voice, a recommendation other than individual or group therapy may be indicated. If the primary problem is decreased volume, the use of an amplification device (portable microphone) may help to improve the voice so that others can better understand what the patient says. In order to spare patients disappointment and undue expense, it is strongly advised that a qualified speech pathologist be consulted before purchasing the voice amplifier. Patients who demonstrate slurred speech, uneven rate, or lack of voice inflection, are unlikely to benefit from amplification; quite the contrary, an amplifier may only exaggerate these problems. Its use can only increase the loudness of the voice; it cannot improve general speech clarity. If, on the other hand, a speech pathology consultation yields a recommendation that such a device is warranted, the speech-language pathologist can assist in choosing the most appropriate amplifier for the patient's needs and can also offer instruction in its use. Many companies now offer a trial period or a guarantee for any amplifier purchased.

Hearing Loss

Hearing loss can be a factor, but is not a direct result of Parkinson's disease. Some degree of hearing loss is not unusual as the body ages. Whatever the cause may be, a hearing deficit can adversely affect good speaking and listening habits. If the Parkinsonian suspects some difficulty with hearing, a medical doctor may recommend a hearing evaluation by an audiologist. A hearing test may also be warranted for spouses or others if they are having difficulty understanding speech. The problem in communication could be complicated by decreased hearing ability in the listener, rather than some condition related entirely to the Parkinsonian's speech.

HOME EXERCISE PROGRAM

For those patients who live in areas of the country where appropriate support services are unavailable, exercises for facial mobility and facial expression, voice loudness and variation, articulation (pronunciation), and rate of speaking can be practiced at home. These exercises should be part of a daily routine; patients can perform them alone or with the help of a family member or caregiver. Throughout any practice session, it is important to use a mirror to focus attention on the mouth and to be aware of what the lips and tongue are doing while speaking, eating, and swallowing. Developing a keen sense of lip and tongue movements will help to improve awareness. Patients should also pay attention to posture, keeping their shoulders erect but relaxed, and the head in an upright position.

Facial Mobility and Expression

As was previously discussed, Parkinsonians may find that facial expessions require a conscious effort if they are to be successfully accomplished. Generally, those afflicted with Parkinson's disease exhibit faces that are less mobile or expressive; others often misinterpret the characteristic mask-like appearance as fatigue, depression, or disinterest. Patients' spouses have often stated, "He always looks like he's mad at me," while still others say, "She never looks like she's interested in anything anymore." It is not at all unusual that Parkinsonians find themselves unable to laugh at a joke, or they look indifferent during a heart wrenching and emotional situation.

The exercises shown on pages 65 and 66 are just a few that patients can do on their own to increase facial mobility and expression.

Lip and Jaw Exercises

Increasing facial muscle mobility can have a positive effect on facial expression, speech, saliva control, and eating. Firm, controlled lip closure is important in the production of well-formed consonants (nonvowel sounds) and in the ability to hold a firm lip seal for the control of saliva and

Home exercise program: do each exercise 10 times, twice daily

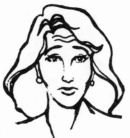

Raise eyebrows—
wrinkle forehead

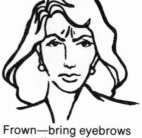

Frown—bring eyebrows
together and down

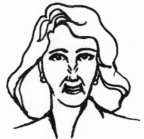

Wrinkle nose—
expression of distaste

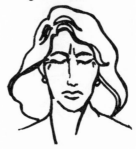

Close eyes tightly

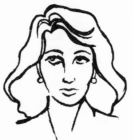

Move both eyes up
& toward the right

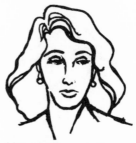

Move both eyes down
& toward the left

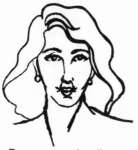

Purse or pucker lips

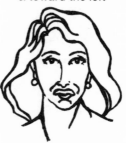

Protrude upper lip

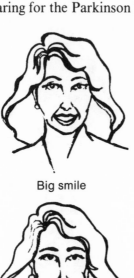

Big smile

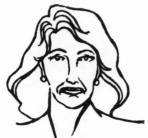

Grimace—draw corners of
your mouth to the sides

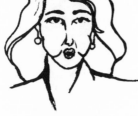

Blow

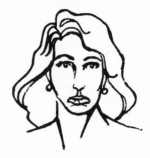

Pout (protrude lower lip)

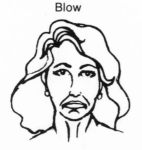

Draw corners of mouth
downward strongly

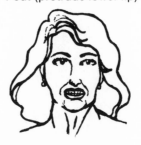

Close jaws tightly

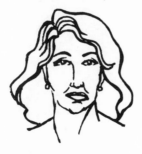

Move jaw forward and
to the side (left and then right)

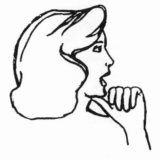

Press jaw down against hand

food during swallowing. The following exercises can help to improve the decreased functioning of muscles in the mouth and jaw:

* Open and close the mouth slowly several times, making sure the lips are closed completely.

* Open the mouth wide, as if saying "ah," then round the lips, as if saying "oo."

* Close the lips and press them together tightly for a few seconds, then relax.

* Alternate rounding the lips and smiling as if saying "oo," then "ee."

* Stretch the lips into a wide smile, hold the tension in the cheek muscles, then relax.

* Puff the cheeks up, hold the air for five seconds, then release it while blowing out.

* Pucker the lips, as for a kiss, hold the tension in the lip muscles, then relax.

* Suck cheeks in, then relax.

* Pucker—Hold. Smile—Hold.

* Let lips flap while blowing air out over them.

* Puff cheeks up with air, then move the air from one cheek to the other without letting it escape.

* Close lips tightly while puffing up the cheeks with air. Hold for five seconds and then release.

Tongue Movements

It is common for there to be less range, less pressure, and less precise movements of the tongue in Parkinsonian patients. If the tongue moves sluggishly, which it often does when attempts are made to speak rapidly, consonant sounds may be indistinct and difficult to distinguish. Strengthening and increasing the range and precision of tongue movements, both for the formation of sounds and for swallowing, can be achieved using the following exercises:

(Use a mirror and do each exercise ten times, twice daily.)

* Stick out your tongue, hold it to feel the tension in the muscles of the tongue, then retract it.

* Elevate the tongue tip, stretching it toward your nose as far as it will go.

* Lower the tip, stretching it toward the chin.

* Rotate your tongue from side to side under the upper lip while holding the lips gently closed.

* Rotate your tongue from side to side under the lower lip while holding the lips gently closed.

* Make a circle with the tongue on the inside of the lips, holding the lips closed.

* Move your tongue from side to side as quickly as possible.

* Stick out your tongue and retract it as quickly as possible.

Suggestions for Practicing Connected Speech

* Make a sentence using the words in this section title.

* Read aloud from a favorite book, magazine, or newspaper.

* Talk with a family member about a specific topic.

Be sure to

* speak slowly,

* exaggerate lip and tongue movements,

* pay particular attention to emphasized word endings,

* limit the number of words spoken in a single breath,

* pause for breath, and

* break up long words into distinct syllables.

Voice Intensity (Loudness) Exercises

Normal speakers pause and take a quick breath between phrases, sentences, and thoughts. In Parkinson's disease the reduction in control and movement of the respiratory muscles requires more frequent breath pauses between words. Parkinsonian patients must learn to pace themselves and pause frequently for breath, otherwise speech volume fades. Exercises can be performed to heighten awareness of the need to increase the frequency of breath intake and to limit the number of words spoken in a single breath.

* Awareness of the inhaling/exhaling rhythm needed for speech can be developed by placing one's hands on the rib cage and then on one's stomach while breathing in and out.

* Coordinate breathing with speech

  Goal: To hold a sound for 15–20 seconds

  > Learn to recognize that a breath is needed if your voice fades. Stop and start again.

Breathe in, say "ah" while exhaling.

Breath in, say "o" while exhaling,

Breath in, say "ee" while exhaling,

Breathe in, say "aw" while exhaling,

Breathe in, say "oo" while exhaling,

  Goal: To maintain loudness and to hold volume without fading

  > Push out more air to achieve loudness.

  > Recognize your limit; take a breath and start again.

Breathe in, say "one."

Breathe in, say "one," "two."

Breathe in, say "one," "two," "three."

Breathe in, say "one," "two," "three," "four."

Breathe in, say "one," "two," "three," "four," "five."

Continue sequence.

Breathe in, say "a."

Breathe in, say "a," "b."

Breathe in, say "a," "b," "c."

Breathe in, say "a," "b," "c," "d."

Breathe in, say "a," "b," "c," "d," "e."

continue sequence.

Goal: To build loudness gradually, soft to loud

Use three levels of loudness.

Push out more air to achieve loudness.

SOFTLY	*LOUDER*	***VERY LOUD***
Be quiet.	*Be quiet.*	***Be quiet!***
Thank you.	*Thank you.*	***Thank you!***
Here.	*Here.*	***Here!***
I'm coming.	*I'm coming.*	***I'm coming!***
Don't do that.	*Don't do that.*	***Don't do that!***
Sit down.	*Sit down.*	***Sit down!***

Voice Inflection (Variation)

Key words in a sentence can be stressed to clarify meaning. Word stress can both change the intent and help to emphasize one's point. Question forms are usually said with an upward tone. Emotion is also conveyed by lowering and raising the volume and stress of certain words. The following exercises should prove helpful:

Goal: To change word stress to achieve a different meaning

Emphasize the italicized word.

I don't want it now.

I *don't* want it now.

I don't *want* it now.

I don't want *it* now.

I don't want it *now*.

Raise and lower your voice as indicated by the arrows.

Are you *going*? ↑

Have you *seen* it? ↑

Can you *do* it? ↑

Is it *yours*? ↑

Did you *know* that? ↑

Do it *now*. ↓

This is *it*. ↓

Sit *down*. ↓

Turn *here*. ↓

Call her *today*. ↓

Speech Improvement Exercises

Without the right kind of skilled professional help, improving speech clarity, voice volume, inflection, and rate is difficult. However, a highly motivated individual can achieve some success if a home program is strictly adhered to and patients diligently strive to apply the strategies to their conversational speech. A home program is designed to stimulate the most efficient use of the speech musculature and to help general intelligibility. Patients should practice regularly each day. They can work alone or with someone who can provide a model and feedback if this is preferred. (See the Appendix at the end of this chapter for additional speech improvement exercises that Parkinsonian patients can practice at home.)

Drill for "f"

Put upper teeth over lower lip and blow air out over lip.

fine	coffee	wife
first	after	knife
feet	sofa	half
find	often	stuff
five	offer	cuff

Drill for "v"

Put upper teeth over lower lip and blow air out over lip as the vocal cords vibrate.

very	oven	love
visit	ever	dive
value	driver	have
voice	even	live
vacation	never	leave

NONVERBAL COMMUNICATION

If patients who suffer from Parkinson's disease are unable to participate in therapy programs because of poor physical stamina or as a result of having reached the advanced stages of the disease, it may be necessary for the speech-language pathologist to discuss with the family and/or caregiver some alternative means of communication. There are nonverbal communication methods used to supplement or substitute for the spoken word when verbal communication has become severely impaired. The effect of these particular methods will be limited if there are other impairments such as severe visual deficits or limited use of the arms and fingers. However, if no physical or educational deficiences exist, the use of nonverbal communication can provide a means of expressing needs and desires.

Communication Charts

The following communication charts are recommended for severely speech impaired individuals who cannot communicate orally or in writing, but can understand spoken or written language. It is important that patients be encouraged to convey basic desires and feelings in a simple nonverbal way.

* Letter Chart: (The patient spells words by pointing to letters.)

* Individual Letter Tiles: (The patient makes words with letter tiles, much like a game of Scrabble®.)

* Word Chart: (The patient points to words.) The words chosen for a word chart should be highly significant for the individual and should include family names, the names of close friends, and words centering around physical comfort and physical needs. The enclosed list includes appropriate word choices.

yes	no	doctor
cold	pain	medication
hot	blanket	water
outside	hungry	bathroom
clothes	get up	wheelchair
eat	sleep	bath
bed	sit	stand
walk	radio	book
TV	eyeglasses	drink

* Picture Chart: (The patient points to pictures.) This technique is used more frequently by those whose physical condition and stamina restrict the use of the letter or word chart.

Communication charts should fit patient requirements and include word and picture choices most significant to the persons who will be using them. It is best to start off with a basic word or picture chart and expand or alter it as speakers and listeners become more adept at using it. The success of using a communication chart is a combined effort, dependent only on the patients' abilities and imagination, understanding, and the patience of listeners.

SUGGESTIONS FOR IMPROVED COMMUNICATION

It is important for emotional well-being and for the management of day-to-day living that Parkinsonian patients not give in to withdrawal and self-imposed isolation because speech has become more difficult. To speak clearly, however, may take conscious effort and a sincere commitment on the patients' part if they are to make their needs, feelings, and thoughts known to others.

Ideas may need to be expressed in short, concise sentences that are more easily understood by listeners. Do not yield to the pressure to answer quickly. Patients should give themselves time to think and to plan what they wish to say and take additional time to speak slowly and clearly. Listeners are to be faced as the pronunciation of each word is exaggerated. Patients should speak as if their listeners are hard of hearing and need to read lips. A breath should be taken before speaking and a pause between every few words, or even between each word. Most important, patients should talk for themselves. Others cannot be permitted to speak for them. Loved ones may have to be reminded not to interrupt or finish patients' sentences. Gestures can be used to facilitate communication. Patients should make a conscious effort to exaggerate facial expressions to provide more cues to listeners about how they are feeling. Care must be taken not to give in to feelings of embarrassment or frustration. Family and friends need the Parkinsonian patient to be an important part of their lives and will assist the patient's efforts to be understood.

APPENDIX

ARTICULATION (PRONUNCIATION) EXERCISES

(Use a mirror and exaggerate lip and tongue movements.)

Drill for "m"

Press lips together firmly,

morning	summer	home
money	stomach	name
Monday	timing	dime
move	hamburger	room
match	coming	some

Drill for "p"

Close lips, puff cheeks up with air, then release.

pie	apple	tip
pills	open	soap
piece	happy	wipe
pull	supper	rope
pencil	copper	nap

Drill for "b"

Press lips together, puff up the cheeks with air, letting the air explode as the vocal cords vibrate.

better	ruby	tab
back	table	knob
because	elbow	fib
bad	able	cab
bed	garbage	tub

Drill for "w"

Round lips as if saying "oo."

way	awake	how
wait	showing	know
water	lower	chew
won	flower	low
was	away	new

Drill for voiceless "th"

Stick tongue out between teeth and blow.

think	birthday	with
thumb	anything	both
three	something	mouth

| thousand | nothing | bath |
| thought | bathtub | north |

Drill for voiced "th"

Stick tongue out between teeth and blow as the vocal cords vibrate.

the	brother	breathe
that	other	smooth
this	another	bathe
those	mother	clothe
then	father	soothe

Drill for "t"

Place the tongue behind the upper teeth and let air pressure explode as the tongue tip is lowered.

time	letter	not
tell	heater	late
talk	enter	hurt
table	lottery	dirt
today	debtor	wait

Drill for "d"

Put the tongue behind the upper teeth and build pressure at the tongue tip.

do	loading	need
day	reading	side
down	ladder	ride
door	adding	food
done	ready	bed

Drill for "n"

Put the tongue behind the upper teeth and let air come through the nose.

now	funny	man
name	many	line
night	sunny	fine
not	running	sun
noisy	honey	one

Drill for "l"

Put the tongue behind the upper teeth as the vocal cords vibrate.

late	alone	tall
let	below	will
laugh	yellow	ball
lady	jello	well
lately	only	hall

Practice tongue elevation in combination with another consonant.

please	black	flat	clean	glad
place	blow	flavor	close	glass
pleasure	blood	flight	clip	glue
plus	blanket	fly	cloudy	glow
plaid	blue	floor	clock	gloves

Drill for "r"

Round the lips slightly and curl the tongue tip back.

ready	sorry	more
ring	carrot	tire
room	borrow	care
right	hurry	hair
rub	carry	fair

Combine the "r" with another consonant.

practice	trap	drive	brag
pray	trouble	drip	broom

pretty	try	drab	brother
promise	trip	dream	brim
predict	truck	dress	brawl

craft	greet	fry
crowd	grasp	fruit
crest	ground	fried
cream	great	fresh
creep	group	frame

Drill for "s"

The lips are smiling as the tongue tip is raised and air is blown down the center of the mouth.

said	beside	mess
soup	outside	house
see	mister	lease
so	lesson	pass
soon	eraser	horse

Practice "s" in combination with another consonant.

smart	sneeze	spell	stay
small	sniff	speak	stop
smoke	snap	spot	star

swim	slow	splash	spray
swing	sleep	split	spread
sweep	slice	splatter	sprinkle

straw	square	scratch
strap	squeak	scream
strike	squint	scribble

Drill for "z"

The lips are smiling as the tongue tip is raised and air is blown down the center of the mouth as the vocal cords vibrate.

zipper	lazy	sneeze
zone	razor	is
zero	dozen	has
zoo	crazy	please
zebra	dizzy	because

Drill for "sh"

Round lips, while raising the sides of the tongue to the upper teeth and blow air out the center of the mouth.

shop	washing	rash
sharp	wishing	rush
shoe	dishes	cash
shine	fishing	bush
should	cushion	push

Drill for "ch"

Raise the sides of the tongue, round the lips and explode air.

cheese	butcher	beach
children	kitchen	catch
chicken	matches	lunch
change	ketchup	reach
chair	teacher	much

Drill for "j"

Round lips and raise tongue to ridge behind upper teeth as the vocal cords vibrate.

just	major	large
jelly	edge	orange

jar	bridges	page
juice	agent	badge
jacket	engine	huge

Drill for "k"

Raise back of tongue as you let air explode.

keep	okay	take
kind	baking	book
key	looking	pick
cold	pocket	work
car	making	make

Drill for "g"

Raise back of tongue, letting air explode as the vocal cords vibrate.

get	begin	egg
go	forgive	tag
good	forget	leg
give	foggy	bag
goad	began	rug

Drill for "h"

Open mouth and exhale.

how	ahead
his	perhaps
hand	anyhow
happy	behind
hurt	unhook

6

Physical Therapy

Jim R. Carpenter

The loss of agility and mobility are distressing features of Parkinson's disease. Through the development of a tailored exercise program and with disciplined adherence to the exercise regime, Parkinsonian patients may anticipate improved functioning. Physical maintenance and/or improvement, however, is not accomplished without combined efforts on the part of the patients, their families, and the health care team.

A medication regime addresses Parkinsonian patients' signs and symptoms; yet it does not directly address secondary musculoskeletal changes, including disuse atrophy, tissue shrinkage, and generalized disability. Well thought out, individualized exercise programs can address these secondary effects and allow patients to maintain maximum mobility.

ASSESSMENT

The physical therapist, in order to develop an effective management program, must examine the patients to determine the extent of structural, functional abnormalities. The examination often reveals common signs of Parkinson's disease: resting tremor, rigidity, akinesia-bradykinesia, and postural reflex (poor balance). These factors often lead to such problems as abnormal body movement, faulty posture and balance, and an altered gait. In many cases, patients will experience great difficulty in moving their limbs whether sitting or standing.

Patients with advanced Parkinson's disease may have difficulty initiating movement and may appear to be in a frozen state. This freezing response may be brought on by minor obstacles. Even the presence of a line painted on the floor could cause patients to freeze during walking. Corners, doorways, hallways, and closets commonly provide difficult obstacles, which result in freezing.

Patients also may have disturbed balance, which leads to falls and causes them to walk with understandable trepidation. Some patients may walk with their weight distributed too far forward; this results in rapid, uncontrolled shuffling, which has been called a festinating gait. The loss of balance is also evident when the patients try to back up to a bed or a chair. They might lose their balance and be propelled backward. This is known as retropulsive gait.

Once the extent of the physical deficits are determined, the physical therapist, with the help of input from the patients, families, physicians, and related health professionals, should be able to develop realistic goals from which a plan of action can be developed. For goals to be realistic, they must be agreed upon by all parties involved.

GOALS

Individualized goals frequently include the following:

1. restoration of a more normal body alignment (posture)
2. enhancement of automatic responses, including balance
3. enhancement of patients' ability to:
   a. initiate movement
   b. move rhythmically
   c. move in normal patterns
   d. ambulate (walk)

A plan of action will involve specific exercises and ambulation routines. These routines should attack specific problem areas and be designed as much as possible to duplicate movement patterns utilized everyday. The activities and the exercise program should reinforce each other to provide optimal carry-over from the exercises to the desired result. Patients, in cooperation with their families, should be encouraged to perform as many of these normal activities as possible, including those involved in personal hygiene. Some patients, because of their disability, will find these activities

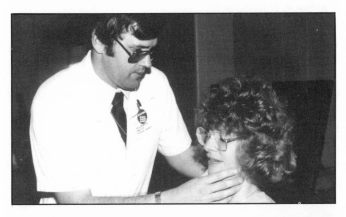

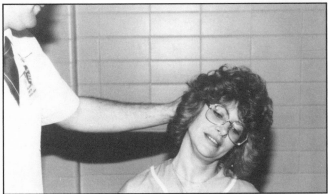

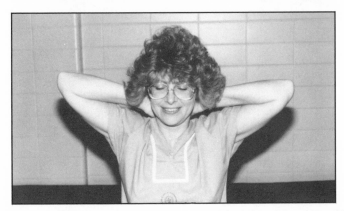

Figure 1. Chin tucks are achieved by stretching the chin out and then "tucking" the chin. Neck side bends are accomplished by bending the neck to each side, stretching the neck muscles. Rolling the shoulders forward and then backward is also beneficial.

extremely tedious. It may be desirable for them to rise early in the morning hours in order to have sufficient time to complete these routines.

The concept of pride in independence must be reestablished for these Parkinsonian patients. Furthermore, in my clinical experience, the patients' levels of activity appear to have a cumulative effect. The more patients exercise on one day, the easier it is for them to do so the next. Conversely, if patients have a period of relative inactivity, their physical capabilities will often regress. The actual number of exercises or ambulation routines, however, should be kept to a minimum. Patients, when confronted with an impressive number of routines, often become overwhelmed; as a result, they do not comply with any of the exercises offered.

TREATMENT PROGRAM

The following section will list predetermined goals, followed by a plan of action that includes examples of specific exercises designed to meet those goals.

Goal I: Restoration of a more normal body alignment and posture

As a result of immobility and the disease process itself, many Parkinsonian patients develop stooped posture flexion contracture involving the neck, back, shoulders, hips, and knees. Both passive and active stretching exercises are needed to regain the normal muscle elongation and to maintain trunk mobility for a satisfactory breathing pattern.

The stretching routines may initially require the assistance of a health professional or a member of the family. Yet, patients should eventually be able to assume responsibility for themselves in this area. The exercise should always be performed gently to allow the muscles to relax slowly and to stretch. Many patients will experience a unique type of muscular stiffness called cogwheel or lead pipe rigidity, which will provide resistance throughout the range of motion. The presence of this rigidity makes the stretching procedures all the more important. Chin tucks, side bends, shoulder rolls, and buttock tucks are all useful stretching exercises, as demonstrated in figure 1 (see p. 83).

The combined effects of trunk immobility, faulty posture, and generalized weakness inhibit adequate rib and trunk movement. These contribute to poor breathing patterns. In order to help regain satisfactory trunk movement, the following exercise example is suggested. Patients,

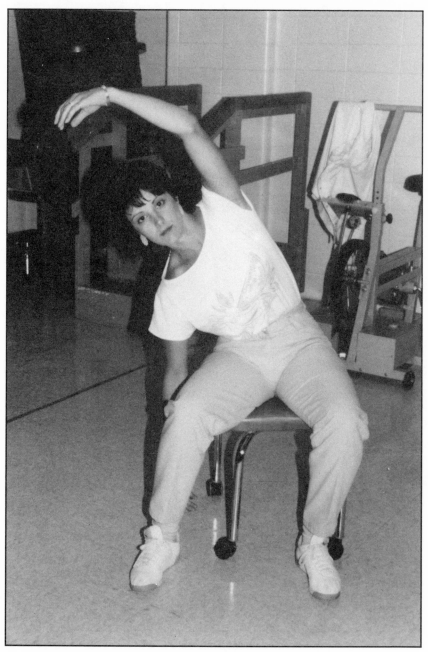

Figure 2. Stretch right arm over head and to the left side as far as possible. Then stretch to the right side.

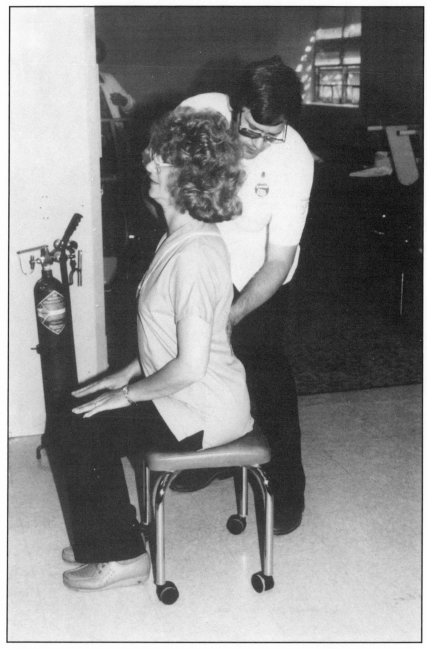

Figure 3. Maintaining correct posture is very important! A slight curve in the lower back, shoulders pulled back, and chin held up will help prevent the stooping that sometimes occurs with Parkinson's disease.

while sitting on a stool, will side-bend as far as possible, first to one, and then to the other side. The side-bending is combined with breathing from the diaphragm. Patients will exhale as they bend toward the floor and inhale as they return to the upright position (see figure 2, p. 85).

It is important that patients become aware of their faulty posture and attempt to correct it. Patients should practice developing a slight arching curve, not only in the neck, but in the lower back as well (see figure 3, p. 86). A lumbar roll, which fits in the curve of the back, or a postural seat cushion is often helpful in this regard.

Goal II: Enhancement of automatic responses, including balance

Patients will require exercises designed to enhance their ability to transfer weight from one leg to the other, combined with all important head and trunk movements (i.e., rotation against the force of gravity). Rotation movements are counter-movements that restore a threatened balance from alterations to the center of gravity. For example, when a sitting patient is pushed to the right, his head and upper trunk quickly rotate to the left, thereby maintaining his center of gravity and his sitting balance. I have used the up and down movement of a tilt table in order to enhance patients' postural reactions through possible stimulations of the semicircular canals of the inner ear. Other clinicians have described routines that utilize equipment such as a vestibular board. Patients are placed either sitting or lying prone on elbows and slowly rocked back and forth. This often has a beneficial effect, with an immediate improvement in automatic response and balance reactions, sometimes for extended periods. Other clinicians have reported the use of a piano stool, by which sitting patients were slowly rotated first in one direction and then the other (see figure 4, p. 88).

Goal III: An enhancement of the patients' ability to

    a. initiate movement

    b. move rhythmically in a reciprocal fashion

    c. move in normal patterns

    d. ambulate

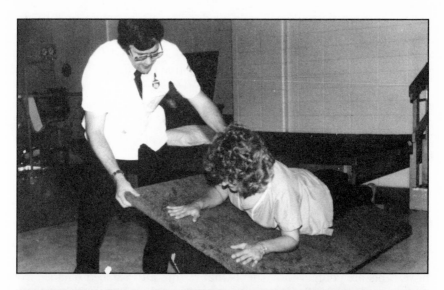

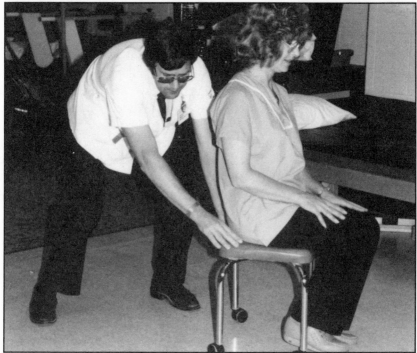

Figure 4. A vestibular board may help improve balance. Rotating while sitting on a piano stool is something the patient might practice at home with the assistance of a family member.

   This goal can be accomplished in a variety of ways. One technique, called *rhythmic initiation,* has been shown to be of value for this problem of movement initiation. The therapist may assist sitting patients in transferring weight forward and backward. This alternately flexes and extends the patients' hips in a rhythmic manner. Gradually, patients progress to a standing position (see figure 5, below). This initiation procedure may also be carried out while patients are lying on their side, thus facilitating rolling. Gradually, patients may be able to initiate these movements on their own.

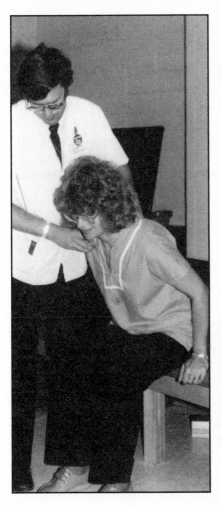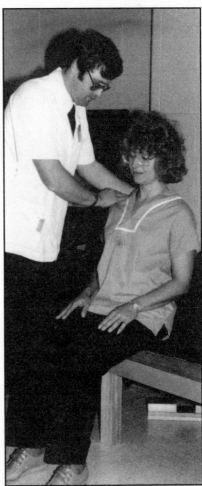

Figure 5. The patient is assisted in leaning forward and then rocking backwards to practice shifting weight to facilitate standing and more normal movement patterns.

Additionally, rhythmic and reciprocal movements are often improved by activities such as cycling, mat activities (rolling, creeping), and alternating movements (see figure 6, below).

Patients may sit with their hands and forearms resting on their laps and then alternately rotate their forearms (palms up, then palms down). The lower extremities might benefit from heel-toe rising, using a similiar method (see figure 7, p. 91).

Ambulation Skills

Many of the problems experienced by Parkinsonian patients become obvious as they attempt to stand and walk. These activities require the body to move in a rhythmic and bilateral fashion incorporating many large muscle groups. There are several types of gait problems, including the patients' cadence, stride, counter-rotation (balance), and propulsion.

Cadence: To improve patients' cadence, stride, and overall freedom of movement, the use of emphasized words, such as counting or singing, either by the patients or their therapist may facilitate smooth movement. Background music has also been proved to be of moderate benefit in many cases. Instructing patients to "march" rather than "just walk naturally" is suggested.

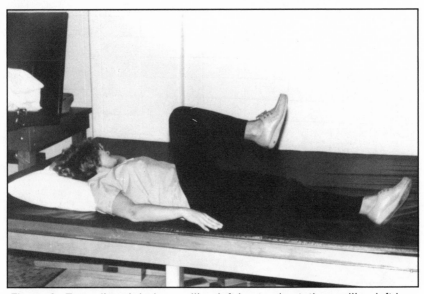

Figure 6. Extending right leg, pulling left leg to chest, then rolling left leg to right side of body; repeat using other leg to improve rhythmic and reciprocal movements.

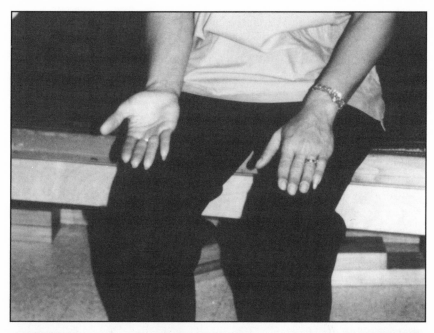

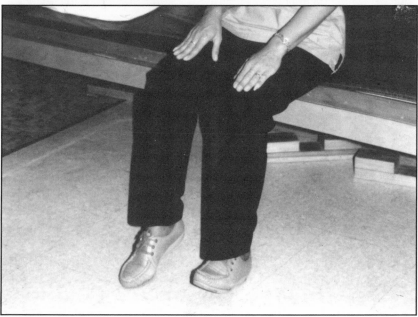

Figure 7. Rotate forearms by turning palm up and then down; also while in a sitting position, practice lifting the heel of your foot up and then down.

Walking may be further enhanced by the use of obstacles that require patients to alter their stride or gait sequence. Included may be routines that make use of equipment such as a foot placement ladder, pieces of paper shaped in the form of footprints, or even tape placed at intervals on the floor. These are all used to stimulate a larger stride. One therapist has advocated fixing a transverse metal bar to the bottom of a cane, over which patients would step (see figure 8, p. 93).

The common denominator for all these gait-assisted devices may be that they require patients to abandon a regular or automatic gait pattern; in so doing, gait becomes more consciously and voluntarily controlled.

Counter-Rotation (balance): Balance, or the lack of it, is the next great concern of the physical therapist. The patients' entire body should be incorporated into the gait pattern in order to provide satisfactory balance reactions. There are various methods that appear to enhance these reactions. For example, patients are instructed to stand facing a wall or door, their arms at shoulder height with elbows extended. They will then rotate one arm, following the movement with their eyes and head, and then alternate to the opposite side. Another example might be for standing patients to squat, rotating their pelvis, while at the same time, rotating their upper trunk to the opposite side (see figure 9, p. 94).

The therapist may choose to assist with the development of arm swing, and thus enhance counter-rotation. A therapist and his patient face each other, each grasping the other's shoulders. The therapist then manually counter-rotates the patient's upper trunk as they both begin to walk. Thus, an arm-swing pattern is duplicated. Broomsticks, canes, and wands have all been utilized to assist manually with this goal (see figure 10, p. 95).

Turns can prove to be very difficult. Patients should be instructed to walk in a circular fashion and never allow their feet to pivot on the ground. Sharp, quick turns and crossing one leg over the other are avoided (see figure 11, p. 96).

Propulsion: Propulsion is yet another common problem that may be helped by a physical therapist. A majority of patients, partly because of their fixed posture, will allow their center of gravity to extend too far forward. As a result, they demonstrate a tendency to walk in short, shuffling steps that often increase in rate. Furthermore, once they are able to initiate gait, they have difficulty stopping. This condition is often helped by the use of negative heel shoes, and by reminding patients to initiate each step by striking their heels to the floor; this keeps the center of gravity directly over the pelvic region.

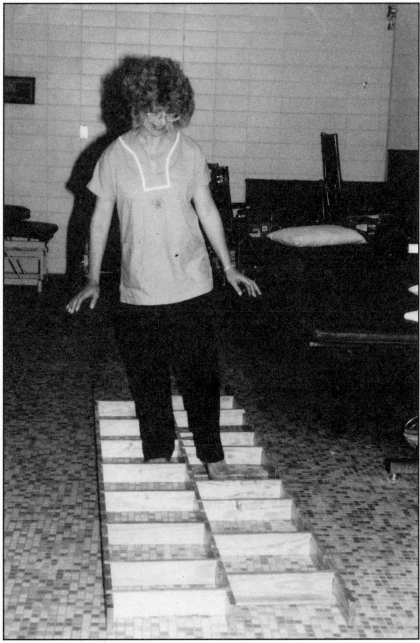

Figure 8. A foot placement ladder may assist in developing a larger stride.

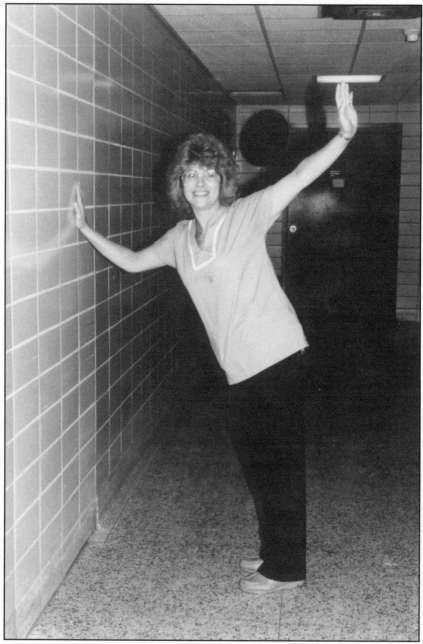

Figure 9. Stand facing the wall; stretch an arm out and around, following its movement with your eyes and head.

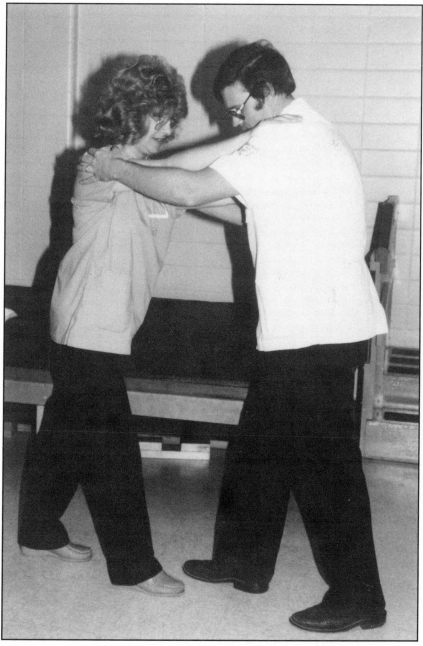

Figure 10. Grasp the patient's shoulder, then rotate patient's upper torso as you both walk to develop a more normal arm swing pattern.

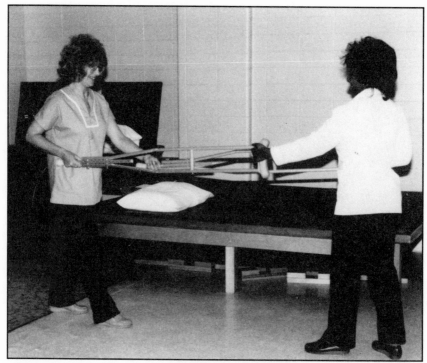

Figure 11. Arm swings can be enhanced by using tools such as a broomstick or crutch to assist the patient in swinging his arms.

CONCLUSION

The reader has been given an overview of the multiple problems often seen in patients afflicted with Parkinson's disease, and the types of treatment routines that have proved beneficial. Patients are encouraged to consult a physical therapist to develop an exercise program individually tailored to their unique needs. Well-motivated patients who carry out the prescribed exercises and gait routines in a persistent fashion will certainly enjoy improvement in physical function, experience an increased feeling of well-being, and enhance their chances of remaining independent.

SUGGESTED READINGS

Brenner, H. J. *Therapeutic Exercises for the Treatment of the Neurologically Disabled.* Springfield, Ill.: Charles C. Thomas, 1957.

Carr, J. H., and Shepherd, R. B. *Physiotherapy in Disorders of the Brain.* London: William Heizemann Medical Books Limited, 1980.

McDowell, F., and Sweet, R. *Manual for Patients with Parkinson's Disease.* The American Parkinson's Disease Association.

7

Falls: A Serious Problem

Carolyn E. Marshall

Falls constitute a very real and serious problem for some persons with Parkinson's disease. From the very first stages of the disease, bodily changes in posture and movement may be noticed by family and friends, sometimes even before the diagnosis has been made.

Even if a disease process such as Parkinson's is not present, falls are a major cause of injuries resulting in impaired mobility. In Great Britain and the United States the incidence of falls among persons over age sixty-five is about 35 to 40 percent, and the risk increases dramatically with advancing age. Less that 20 percent of falls among those aged sixty-five and over are considered serious, and only 6 percent of injurious falls result in fracture, but elderly persons who do fall, and who repeatedly fall as they grow older, account for the major portion of traumatic illness, disability, and death over age sixty-five. The Mayo Clinic estimates that in this age group the cost of medical care nationally for acutely ill patients with hip fracture is in excess of $1 billion per year.

For those 6 percent of falls that do result in fracture, extended immobilization is often the result; pneumonia is a frequent complication that can be life-threatening. Between 1945 and 1980, persons over age sixty-five accounted for approximately 75 percent of home injury deaths associated with falls. All investigators agree that in this age group the overwhelming number of falls occur in the home. Persons with Parkinson's disease are likely to account for an increasing number of these falls because they spend more and more time in the home as the disease progresses.

Older people are at risk of falling under circumstances in which younger people would not fall, perhaps because of lessening postural control or adaptability, or the effects of medications. The individual with Parkinson's disease fits into all of these categories. Postural sway and an unsteadiness of the body during quiet standing increases markedly in some persons past the age of sixty-five. Postural sway is more common among females than males. It has been proposed that the normally lighter musculature of females could be the cause. Over time, women fall twice as much as their male counterparts, and the falls are more likely to recur.

Mobility and independence are intertwined. The former can be defined as the ability to function satisfactorily in the home or in the community. Even if no injury results, a fall often prompts individuals who function independently to limit their activity because of a deep-seated fear that they may fall again and sustain injury. This reduced activity can be the beginning of a downward spiral that is all too common in Parkinsonian patients. They can easily slip into a cycle of moving only from the bed to a chair to the kitchen or bathroom and back to bed, all the while losing strength and coordination. Social and mental stimulation diminish and feelings of isolation and depression are common. Now the stage is set for the self-fulfilling prophesy of another fall, perhaps this time with injury and loss of mobility and independence. Many older persons lose their independence as a result of being unable to function in their home environments. Either the elderly themselves or their families/caregivers believe them to be at risk of falling and may unnecessarily restrict important opportunities for social interaction and independent functioning.

Just as Parkinsonism initially appears in different individuals at different ages, it moves through its five stages (see chapter 1) at different rates, and balance is affected along the way. Stage 1 is a mild form of the disease that affects only one side of the body and typically persists for a year or two before becoming bilateral. As patients stand and move about, they may hold an affected arm in a semiflexed position and lean to the unaffected side; this alone can affect balance and an increased tendency to fall.

Stage 2 demonstrates bilateral involvement and may show noticeable postural changes. Patients tend to assume a stooped posture when standing or walking, often with a slow, shuffling gait. Falls caused by tripping may begin to occur because the feet are not raised in a normal manner when walking. The simple combination of a high napped carpet and crepe-soled shoes can cause trips and falls. Bradykinesia develops and patients may complain of tiredness and lethargy. Reduced mobility may include problems in starting to walk and sudden, abrupt freezing of muscles once movement has been initiated. Balance can be affected by a decrease in natural arm swing or the short, shuffling steps known as festination. Parkinsonian patients who experience difficulty with walking and balance may, at times, resemble a moving car without brakes.

Stage 3 has pronounced balance disturbances along with the onset of gait retropulsion and propulsion. Entering a closet or a narrow hall where patients have to back up to exit can create panic because patients know that they need space to negotiate a broad-based turn in order to reverse direction without losing balance. If that space is not available, attempting to move backward often results in a loss of balance and a fall. Retropulsion becomes a very real problem in daily life when an individual attempts a simple activity such as stepping backward to open the door of a refrigerator or car. The progressively faster and smaller steps of propulsion find the patients' trunk inclined forward farther and farther until a fall occurs. Some Parkinsonians begin to accept more and more help because of fatigue and slowness, while others refuse most assistance with fierce determination.

Stage 4 is marked by significant disability as patients need more and more help with daily activities and almost constant supervision. Rigidity and bradykinesia make all movement slow and uncertain. Rising from a sitting position and turning over in bed are difficult; a slight push will send a standing individual into severe retropulsion or propulsion and will most likely result in a fall.

When Stage 5 is fully developed, the patients are total invalids. Parkinson's disease begins insidiously and pursues a slow and progressive course for fifteen to twenty years or longer. There is considerable variability in progression from stage to stage and from individual to individual.

When falls begin to occur, both patients and family members need to weigh the risks involved against the patients' continued independence. As the disease progresses, alterations in decisions may need to occur. Matteson has pointed out that humans do not normally exist in a risk free environment. A tenuous balance is struck between an environment that is sufficiently challenging to promote growth and skill development and one that is potentially hazardous. If restrictions are placed on an individual's activity in the hope of preventing falls, risk of injury due to disuse atrophy is a possibility. As activity is restricted, limited competence becomes further compromised so that a fall is now more likely to occur, and, if it does, the possibility of injury from the fall is enhanced. The question of costs and benefits to those concerned must be weighed. Is the price of added protection worth it? It depends on the individuals involved and their respective values. Protection against injury, like drug therapy, must be tailored to the individual; it seldom involves interventions with no adverse effects. Both patients and caregivers must be part of the decision making.

CASE HISTORY 1*

The long marriage of Dr. and Mrs. Smith has included life in the military, travel, and an active social life both in the community and in the university. Mrs. Smith was diagnosed as having Parkinson's disease about four years ago; its progression has been rapid and she is very sensitive to the medications, though she is part of the experimental drug program. Both say that each supports the other and that the strength of their marriage has been reinforced as the disease progresses; Dr. Smith is always alert for his wife's nonverbal signals that she needs aid.

Mrs. Smith's first major fall resulted in a hip fracture that isolated her for over a year. Although she does not consider herself a frequent faller, she cannot get up unaided after a fall. Her particular body build and the tendency of women to sway more as they age because of lighter musculature may be a factor in this, but it is a frequently reported result of Parkinson's disease. Mrs. Smith willingly accepts help from her husband. Both are very comfortable with the fact that she will call when she is in need; interdependence and mutual support have been integral parts of their long married life. Mrs. Smith feels that it may be more difficult for a man to slow down and be careful or to ask for help. They walk together for exercise.

Mrs. Smith's hip fracture occurred when she tried to push an object; she knew she should never try to push, pull, or pick up anything, no matter how small or light, if there was a chance it would throw her off balance. She was trying to help her husband load a trailer at a time when they were under pressure to meet a commitment. Even though it was early in the progression of the disease, her balance was impaired.

She reports that increasing stiffness in her neck and shoulders means that now she can no longer simply turn her head, but must turn her whole body; if she is standing or walking, this often means she will lose her balance and fall. Each movement must be carefully calculated. She tries to be very careful not to reach forward to pick up anything, not even

---

*The names have been changed.

a magazine. A chopping block in the middle of the kitchen helps her keep her balance while cooking. Moving too close to the counter or sink means that her feet may become "stuck" and she is unable to move away unless she has something, or someone, to hold onto to help maintain her balance.

After falling in the closet several times and becoming entangled in clothes, shoes, and hangers, Mrs. Smith carefully holds onto the frame of their sliding closet doors to give herself both stability while in the closet and maneuverability when she wishes to exit.

Diminished blinking causes Mrs. Smith to have dry eyes. She also notices a decreased ability to focus; this increases her tendency to fall and also cuts down on her reading (once a great pleasure) expecially when combined with a decreased ability to hold a book because of her diminishing strength.

Mrs. Smith was told that a low protein diet might enhance the effects of her medication. She mistakenly translated this to mean fasting. Within a short time, she had difficulty walking down the hall. She discovered that there are numerous good complex carbohydrates, fruits, and vegetables to substitute for protein in her diet. Thereafter, she was careful to get advice from her physician. Strength and energy need to be maintained, not only to prevent falls, but for general well-being.

The Smiths emphasize that retaining a sense of humor is essential for their situation. Even going to bed requires a positive frame of mind. Mrs. Smith describes how she gets ready for bed with her husband's help and then "dives into bed, all in a heap." Dr. Smith then makes her comfortable by straightening her out and arranging her pillows and covers. During the night, she wakes him up when she needs to turn over or to get up to go to the bathroom. Observation and anticipation of his wife's needs are obviously Dr. Smith's main focus these days. Several times during the interview, he took her unspoken cue and walked across the room to help her straighten up in her chair.

CASE HISTORY 2*

Mr. Jones was diagnosed with Parkinson's disease sixteen years ago at age thirty-nine, when he was a jet fighter pilot. He and his wife admit that he always "lived life in the fast lane." Shifting into a slower gear

---

*The names have been changed.

and into a different position in the military, he retired a few years ago. Mrs. Jones says he gets very impatient when his mind says go and his body says no. As with most couples similarly situated, the Jones state that "they" have Parkinson's disease. They are active in a Parkinson's disease support group and are also in an experimental drug program.

Mr. Jones is a frequent faller and reports three major falls per day with possibly twenty more such instances in which he catches himself. He feels the need to get himself right up as soon as possible and to demonstrate that he is back in control. Mr. Jones is able to get up unaided and rejects his wife's help; he often doesn't let her know he has fallen. He doesn't want to worry her and balks at wearing his "lifeline" device around his neck. He will do this if she is leaving the house for any length of time, if only to give her peace of mind. Swimming is his form of regular exercise.

The mucous that forms on his eyes because of lessened blinking tends to cloud and blur Mr. Jones's vision and contributes to his tendency to trip and fall. He spends time each morning cleaning his eyes with baby shampoo. Falling is such a depressing thing that he says he might be tempted to just go off and hide; however, he simply cannot let himself do that. What is frightening is not the number of times he actually falls, but the number of times he has to catch himself in a single day. Fatigue from loss of sleep the previous night, too much protein for breakfast or lunch, some sort of psychological stress such as a time commitment, or a combination of many small things can cause an individual to have a bad day when falls are more frequent. On such days Mr. Jones believes it may be best not to attempt to take a shower or dress, but to save his energies and assume that tomorrow will be better.

Mr. Jones's falls happen almost instantaneously. He says he has fallen in almost every spot in every room in the house, and only has time to decide where he wants to toss whatever he is carrying. He maintains his humor by saying, "Hey, I'm still in charge here, most of the time." Using a cane at home has cut down on the number of falls, but he says his pride makes him leave it at home when he goes out; he has never figured out just what to do with a cane in a restaurant, for instance. He isn't sure whether a cane is a help or a handicap, but if you feel you need it, you'd better use it! This is part of his effort to balance risk against independence. Mr. Jones makes good use of his cane by using it as a "third foot" with which to maneuver in the closet. He is also experimenting with using it to reach for objects such as a briefcase when he is sitting in a chair.

Mrs. Jones is very supportive of her husband and respects his fierce independence. It is evident that she would like him to be a little less adventurous; in fact, she would like him to use his lifeline signalling device more often. She is very proud of his interest in learning everything he can about Parkinson's disease.

Both couples in these case histories believe that mutual support means a better quality of life for Parkinsonian patients and their families. They find that support exists from within their families and from membership in their local Parkinson's Disease Support Group.

HOME SAFETY

Bathroom Safety

Since most people spend a significant part of their time at home, a discussion of the role that residential architecture plays in falls is in order. The bathroom is the most dangerous room in the house when it comes to slips and falls, so let's look there first and suggest some ways to make it safer and more convenient:

Remove glass shower/tub doors and replace them with a shower curtain.

Keep glass objects out of the bathroom. Paper or plastic cups are safer and more sanitary.

Do not use throw rugs or wax on the bathroom floor.

Watch for water spills on bare floors.

Wall-to-wall carpeting or a room-size rug are the safest forms of floor covering.

A bath chair or stool in the shower/tub will conserve energy and prevent falls.

Grab bars make it easier to get into or out of the shower/tub.

A hand-held shower is sometimes easier to use while seated on the shower stool.

Nonslip strips or a mat in the shower/tub can help to prevent falls.

Soap on a rope or barsoap placed in a nylon stocking with one end tied to a towel bar saves bending over to pick up dropped soap.

A long-handled sponge, bath brush, or wash mitt makes bathing easier.

A nail brush with suction cups attached to the wash bowl makes nail care more convenient.

Electric razors are safer for persons with Parkinson's tremor.

A raised toilet makes sitting and rising easier. Arm rails or a grab bar attached to an adjacent wall work well.

It is smart to make sure someone is within hearing distance when in the bathroom. Don't lock the door! Better yet, leave the door cracked just in case assistance is needed.

A nightlight in the bathroom makes it safer for everyone.

Kitchen Safety

The kitchen has some of the same pitfalls as the bathroom, but here are a few suggestions to make what is arguably the most popular room in the house easier to manage and its decor less hazardous.

Watch for spills that might cause a fall. Keep a long-handled sponge mop handy to wipe them up immediately.

A dustpan attached to a wooden dowel or an old broom handle will allow pick up during sweeping but without the dangers of bending over.

Do not wax a bare floor or use throw rugs; wall-to-wall carpeting is a good choice.

A telephone on the counter is better than one mounted on the wall. If a fall does occur and getting up is not a possibility, pulling the phone off the counter to the floor will allow a call for help. A wall-mounted phone is unreachable.

Frequently used dishes, utensils, and food should be in a convenient spot where reaching is not required.

Wooden reachers, or tongs, are available when it is necessary to reach for light objects.

Lazy Susans used as cabinet organizers or on table or counter tops reduce the need for reaching.

A crock pot will eliminate the need to bend over and put in or remove heavy objects from the oven.

Tables and chairs with casters will roll and cause a loss of balance; remove all casters!

Stair and Carpet Safety

If stairs are an inevitable part of the environment, make them as safe to use as possible by installing handrails on both sides.

Stairs should be well lighted, with switches at both the top and the bottom.

If stairs are carpeted, make sure carpeting is short napped and secure. If they are bare, make sure they are not slippery.

Thresholds at interior doors and inclines, such as ramps, can cause trips and falls from loss of balance. Be very cautious.

Carpeting should have short nap and a tight twist.

Crepe-soled shoes can cause trips and falls from the toes catching in the carpet.

Door Safety

Pulling or pushing on heavy interior or exterior doors, or doors with automatic openers that work too quickly, can cause loss of balance.

Levers are easier to use than door knobs.

Lighting Considerations

The lighting levels should be as consistent as possible throughout the house to avoid false perceptions and confusion about floor levels, especially in a situation where there is a step up or a step down into the next room.

Sun glare onto floor surfaces can cause confusion and loss of balance. Use sheer curtains to admit light without glare.

Furniture Considerations

Chairs and sofas that are soft and low are hard to rise from without help. A straight back chair with a firm seat and arms helps in both sitting and rising.

A firm cushion or chair risers can be used to make chairs the correct height. The seat should never be lower than knee height.

Chairs that automatically raise and tilt the seat forward are available and get rave reviews from their owners. (Check with your insurance company. These chairs may be a covered expense.)

WALKING TIPS

The great outdoors will be safer if a cane is used. Uneven ground, cracks in the sidewalk, and curbs are negotiated more easily.

Don't try to hurry when crossing a street.

CONCLUSION

Many of the preceding suggestions are useful in any setting, whether a private home, a retirement center, or a long-term care facility. A Home Assessment Sheet is appended to this chapter to help in identifying situations that may need to be changed.

APPENDIX

HOME ASSESSMENT SHEET

	YES	NO
Are there stairs in the home?	___	___
If yes:		
Is there a handrail on one side?	___	___
on both sides?	___	___
Is there a light switch at the top or bottom?	___	___
at the top and bottom?	___	___
Are stairs well lighted?	___	___
If carpeted, is carpeting secure?	___	___
If bare, are stairs slippery?	___	___
Are stairs in good repair?	___	___
Are floors carpeted?	___	___
If yes:		
Is carpeting well secured?	___	___
Does carpeting have short nap?	___	___
If no:		
Do floors have a nonskid finish?	___	___
Are large area rugs well secured?	___	___
Do small rugs have nonskid backs?	___	___
Are there thresholds at interior doorways?	___	___
Are there any ramps?	___	___
Is there a step stool or step ladder used in the home?	___	___
If yes, is it sturdy?	___	___
Do any chairs or tables have casters?	___	___
Tub/shower combination?	___	___
Stall shower?	___	___
Nonskid surface on bottom of tub or shower?	___	___
Hand grips or rails in bathroom?	___	___
Light switches at all room entrances?	___	___

	YES	NO
Easy to reach bedside lamp?	____	____
Night light for bathroom trips?	____	____
Is lighting uniform?	____	____
Sheer curtains at windows to reduce glare?	____	____
Are entrance doors easy to open and close?	____	____
Is there a step immediately adjacent to entrance door?	____	____

Source: Carolyn Marshall, "Does Architectural Design Affect the Incidence of Falls Among the Aging?" Thesis, The University of Texas Health Sciences Center at Houston School of Public Health, 1985.

SUGGESTED READINGS

Cape, Ronald, T.T. "Falls in the Elderly: Can We Prevent Them?" The University of Texas Health Science Center at San Antonio Library: Video Tape 785: The Network for Continuing Education, New York, 1984.

Duvoisin, Roger. "Clinical Symposia; Parkinsonism." CIBA Pharmaceutical Company, Summit, N.J., 1976.

Grant, Arthur E. "Use It Or Lose It." *Texas Health Letter,* The University of Texas at Houston (Winter 1984–1985).

Lieberman, A.N.; Gopinathan, G.; Neophytides, A.; and Goldstein, M. *Parkinson's Disease Handbook.* (No date.) Available from an American Parkinson's Disease Association Information and Referral Center or its national office, 116 John Street, New York, New York 10038.

Marshall, Carolyn. "Does Architectural Design Affect the Incidence of Falls Among the Aging?" Masters Thesis, The University of Texas Health Science Center at Houston, School of Public Health. Houston, 1985.

Matteson, M. A., and McConnell. E. S. *Gerontological Nursing: Concepts and Practice.* Philadelphia: W. B. Saunders, 1988.

O'Sullivan, S. B.; Cullen, K. E.; and Schmitz, T. J.; *Physical Rehabilitation: Evaluation and Treatment Procedures,* Philadelphia: F. A. Davis, 1988.

Rowe, J. W., and Besdine, R. W.. *Health and Disease in Old Age.* Boston: Little, Brown and Company, 1982.

Wild, Deirdre. "Falls in the Home." *Nursing Times Community Outlook* (November 9, 1983): 320.

8

Coping with Sleep Disturbance

Raye Lynne Dippel and J. Thomas Hutton

Individuals with Parkinson's disease frequently complain of having difficulty falling asleep and staying asleep. The reduced levels of brain monoamines that result in Parkinson symptoms and symptoms of depression also result in sleep disturbances. In a recent study we conducted, disturbed sleep was reported in 40 percent of the Parkinsonian patients, as compared to 11 percent of the spouses who reported disturbances in sleep. The Parkinsonian patients surveyed complained of frequently waking in the night, of sleepiness and fatigue in the daytime, of nonrestorative sleep, and of restless legs when falling asleep. In other studies, patients have been found to fall asleep more slowly and to have shorter durations of sleep than individuals who do not have the disease.

Medications that are commonly used to treat depression and anxiety do not predictably treat or reduce the sleep complaints of Parkinsonian patients. To minimize sleep disturbance, the administration of levodopa might be maximized in the morning and afternoon, and minimized after 6:00 or 7:00 P.M. Levodopa-induced sleep disturbance may be manifested by vivid dreaming and nightmares. Alternatively, some patients with advanced Parkinson's who experience the end of dose "wearing off" phenomenon may awaken severely bradykinetic, rigid, and tremulous, requiring an additional dose of levodopa. Nocturnal myoclonus (sudden muscle jerks) is known to awaken some Parkinsonians. This condition responds to clorazopam.

In many cases, modifying poor sleeping habits can reduce sleep complaints. In contrast to the common belief that elderly persons "need" more sleep, an adult's need for sleep actually declines steadily through the years, from eight or nine hours of sleep to six or less hours of sleep needed by the sixth and seventh decades of life. Older adults frequently go to bed by eight o'clock, and then complain of not being able to go to sleep or of early morning wakening. Perhaps the person is just not sleepy, resulting from naps taken during the day. The perceived need for naps may be due more to boredom and inactivity than to a real "need" for sleep. In many cases, the individual with sleep disturbance may be suffering from too "much" sleep, rather than too little.

BEHAVIORAL MANAGEMENT OF SLEEP DISTURBANCE

Both Parkinsonian patients and aging patients in general who complain of sleep disturbance might benefit from the following suggestions:

1. Go to bed at the same time, whenever possible.

2. Consider delaying bedtime for an hour or two.

3. Awake at the same time every morning, no later than seven o'clock.

4. Afternoon naps should be avoided. Rest periods may be needed, but avoid sleeping.

5. Develop challenging and interesting activities to fill your day. Boredom is not a good reason for going to sleep.

6. Daily exercise is very important. An early evening walk or exercise program should increase wakefulness until an appropriate bedtime when the individual is actually tired.

7. Restrict reading and other activities to places other than the bed. The bed should be reserved for sleeping; it should be a stimulus for sleep, not for wakefulness.

8. If you awake during the night and have difficulty going back to sleep, get up, engage in an activity (e.g., reading, watching television) until you again feel sleepy, then return to bed. In Parkinsonian patients who awaken with bradykinesia and rigidity, walking and stretching may prove useful prior to trying to go back to sleep.

9. Avoid caffeinated beverages after seven o'clock. Enjoy a small snack before going to bed.

10. Some Parkinsonians benefit from a change in sleeping places. Moving from bed to sofa, recliner, or pallet may facilitate going to sleep.

11. Advanced Parkinsonians who awaken in the night with levodopa "wearing-off" effect (increased symptoms of bradykinesia, rigidity, and tremor) usually benefit from an extra dose of levodopa.

12. Parkinsonians who awaken secondary to too much dopaminergic effect (vivid dreaming, hallucination, dyskinesia) may benefit from taking a protein snack. Protein's ability to reduce the transport of levodopa to the brain can be useful in reducing dyskinesia symptoms and effects.

SUGGESTED READING

Miles, L., and Demont, W. "Sleep and Aging." *Sleep* 3 (1980): 1-220.

9

Psychiatric Aspects

Terry McMahon

Since Parkinson's original description of the shaking palsy in 1870, the disease that bears his name has long been recognized as a neurologic illness that can significantly and adversely affect the lives of patients and families. Some estimates suggest that as many as one percent of the U.S. population over age fifty may develop the core syndrome.

While these neurological symptoms are widely recognized and associated with Parkinson's disease, psychiatric symptoms may be less commonly recognized and appreciated. Historically, this phenomenon can be related to several factors. Parkinson himself initially excluded intellectual changes as a part of the syndrome. Likewise, subsequent reports often did not give particular attention to other psychiatric symptoms as a part of this syndrome.

However, reports over the last several decades have documented that a significant number of Parkinsonian patients may manifest prominent psychiatric symptoms. This heightened recognition of psychiatric symptoms may relate to several factors: (1) a general increase in life expectancy, which may allow the disease to develop further and manifest these symptoms; (2) advances in drug therapies, i.e., dopaminergic and anticholinergic agents, which may, in addition to their therapeutic effects, produce significant psychiatric side effects; (3) an increased awareness of how the basic human nervous system may foster changes in behavior, personality, and mood among such patients.

This chapter will attempt to describe the significant psychiatric symptoms that can be associated with Parkinson's disease and will include: (1) psychiatric symptoms prior to and during early phases of Parkinson's disease; (2) psychiatric symptoms associated with the middle and later phases of the disease; and (3) those symptoms that may be side effects of treatment. Finally, I will conclude with some comments regarding the management of these symptoms.

PSYCHIATRIC SYMPTOMS PRIOR TO AND DURING EARLY PHASES

While it is tempting to identify typical predisease personality changes in Parkinsonian patients, a specific change in personality has yet to be identified. In speaking with patients, clinicians have noted a tendency in some patients to be obsessive, reserved, self-critical, inflexible, and socially withdrawn. Such descriptive terms suggest possible psychological and behavioral features that correlate with the neurological picture in which muscular rigidity and reduced movement often become prominent. However, these correlates, even if consistently present, have yet to be linked to neurological conditions associated with Parkinson's disease. Hence, for now, while investigators continue in their attempts to establish the consistency or specificity of these personality and behavioral attributes, we must remain cautious in attributing these changes to the underlying condition of the nervous system.

From a symptomatic standpoint, clinicians have also noted that depression and vague physical complaints (e.g., decreased mood, decreased self-esteem, tiredness, malaise, decreased energy, and minor aches and pains) may be prominent prior to and during early phases of the disease. Such symptoms are often nonspecific and, early on, they may be attributed to poor diet, poor sleeping patterns, or arthritis. However, given these possible associations, the presence of the symptoms may warrant serious consideration of Parkinson's disease in patients who have no prior psychiatric history. This may be particularly important if relatives note any changes in gait, posture, or speech; the patients themselves are often unaware of these subtle neurological changes early in the course of Parkinson's disease.

Finally, it should be noted that levels of awareness may be mildly affected in the early stages of the disorder. Difficulty with responding to shifting ideas while at the same time maintaining general mental acuity has been described in patients in early phases of the disease. These changes have also been linked to the "obsessive" personality features described above.

Again, while specific, reliable findings have yet to be established, reports by families or patients of slowness in thinking, problem solving, or recall of memories—particularly when they coexist with vague physical or neurological symptoms, as noted above—may warrant consideration of Parkinson's disease.

PSYCHIATRIC SYMPTOMS ASSOCIATED WITH THE MIDDLE AND LATER PHASES OF THE DISEASE

The psychiatric syndromes that have been most commonly linked with this phase of Parkinson's disease include depression and dementia. However, in addition, acute psychotic disorders have also been described in a smaller group of patients.

Depression in particular has received increased attention because of research that has explored the neurological and chemical foundations of both depression and Parkinson's disease. Depression has been linked to changes in the central nervous system's ability to process norepinephrine and serotonin (two major kinds of neurotransmitters) while Parkinson's disease has been clearly associated with diminution of dopamine levels in specific areas of the brain. Since the body processes dopamine and norepinephrine in a similar way, it has been tempting to link depression with Parkinson's disease at this neurochemical level. Morever, dopamine depletion itself has been linked in animal models to behavior that would be viewed as a sign of depression if found in humans. However, until further research clarifies the significance of these findings, such relationships must remain hypothetical and speculative.

Estimates of the incidence of depression range from 35 percent to 90 percent in Parkinsonian patients. From a psychiatric perspective, certain aspects deserve specific comment. First, it can be useful to help patients and families differentiate problems with the depressed mood, which may be more transient and reactive to the stress of the illness and it's complications, from a true clinical depression in which the depressed mood is more sustained and accompanied by symptoms such as sleep disturbance (especially early morning awakening), appetite and weight changes, persistent negative or pessimistic ruminations about one's self or situation, lack of mood reactivity, and the presence of suicidal ideas. (These and similar symptoms are often referred to as *neurovegetative syndrome* because it affects the involuntary nervous system that controls body functions and glandular secretions.)

Second, given the overlap between the neurological symptoms of Parkinson's disease per se, and neurovegetative symptoms commonly associated with depression, it may be especially important to focus on the nonphysical features of depression when considering a diagnosis of depression. More specifically, persistent negativism or pessimism, a negative view of self, lack of mood reactivity, and persistent early morning awakening may suggest that a superimposed depression exists that may deserve specific intervention.

Dementia has also been linked to the middle and later phases of Parkinson's disease. As noted by other contributors to this volume (e.g., see chapter 11), dementia may be defined as an acquired degeneration of general intellectual function related to brain dysfunction. Recently, a hypothetical distinction has been proposed between Alzheimer's disease as a so-called "cortical" dementia (localized on the surface or cortex of the brain) and Parkinson's disease as a so-called "subcortical" dementia (associated with an interior area of the brain). In addition to this differentiation based on location of the disease process in the brain, this hypothesis also suggests some differences in symptoms. Whereas Alzheimer's dementia may be characterized by aphasia (disorder of language due to brain dysfunction), amnesia (difficulty with recalling material), agnosia (failure to recognize or identify objects despite intact sensory function), apraxia (inability to carry out motor activities despite comprehension and motor function), and relative freedom from gait and motor dysfunction, subcortical dementia may be characterized more by a relative lack of aphasia, more difficulty in retrieval of learned material (i.e., forgetfulness), slow problem solving, more personality and mood changes (i.e., depression and apathy), and prominent disturbances of gait and motor function.

While Parkinsonian patients in the past were felt to be relatively free of dementia, a significant number of patients (some estimate as many as 20 to 80 percent) now are believed to be presenting symptoms of dementia. It may be especially useful to note that there appears to be a correlation between increased duration and severity of the Parkinson's disease and the severity of the symptoms of dementia.

So-called paroxysmal disorders (sudden attacks of Parkinson's) have also been attributed to the middle and later phases of the disease. These may include acute psychotic episodes with delusions and hallucinations that resemble either mania or schizophrenia, anxiety attacks, episodes (called perseverative episodes) involving a compulsion to perform tasks that involve the repeating of numbers or words, paranoia, and attacks of unusual or bizarre sensations in the extremities. In contrast to depression and dementia, such disturbances are felt to be less common and often abruptly resolve themselves after a short period of time without specific intervention.

PSYCHIATRIC SYMPTOMS RELATED TO DRUG THERAPY

Medications that enhance dopaminergic function (dopaminergic agents such as levodopa, carbidopa, bromocriptine, and amantadine) and medications that diminish cholinergic function (anticholinergic agents such as benzlropine, trihexyphenidyl, and diphenhydramine have been the mainstays of drug therapy in Parkinson's disease. Both of these major groups of medications have also been linked to psychiatric symptoms.

Anticholinergic agents have the potential to produce a variety of psychiatric symptoms. Anticholinergic toxicity may manifest itself through such physical signs and symptoms as fever, hot and dry skin and mucous membranes, dry mouth, dilated pupils, distended abdomen, constipation, and retaining urine in the bladder. In addition, changes in psychiatric/ mental status are often present and include confusion, disorientation, hallucinations (primarily visual), euphoria, and psychomotor agitation. It should be noted that elderly patients may be particularly susceptible to these medications and may be further predisposed as a result of being prescribed several medications with anticholinergic properties. Patients with signs of dementia may also be predisposed to experience the adverse effects of these agents. It should be noted that many antidepressant and antipsychotic medications have these anticholinergic properties and can precipitate these symptoms when used in inappropriate dosages.

Dopamine toxicity can produce a characteristic syndrome including vivid dreams and nightmares, night terrors (characterized by thrashing and calling out during sleep and waking with prominent anxiety and fear without recall of the dream state), hallucinations (auditory and visual), delusions, paranoia, insomnia, elevated or hypomanic mood, and hypersexuality. A large number of the acute psychotic episodes experienced by Parkinsonian patients may be linked to the effect of these dopaminergic medications. More than one third of patients may develop some or all of these symptoms after two or more years of exposure to dopaminergic agents. A progression of such symptoms has also been suggested, beginning with vivid dreams, nightmares and night terrors, then progressing through hallucinatory experiences and paranoia. In particular it should be noted that the duration and severity of the Parkinsonism may also be linked with a tendency toward these reactions and that patients with a prior history of schizophrenia may be susceptible to reexperiencing their psychotic symptoms as a result of exposure to these agents.

ASSESSMENT AND MANAGEMENT
OF PSYCHIATRIC COMPLICATIONS

If Parkinsonian patients develop any of the psychiatric symptoms noted above, a thorough and comprehensive evaluation is certainly warranted. Initially it is appropriate to take a history from the patient or family, which may particularly focus on whether there have been prior episodes or previous treatment for a major psychiatric disorder that could recur in the context of Parkinson's disease. If so, a history of effective treatment, both behavioral and cognitive as well as pharmacologic, should be elicited since these will prove valuable in guiding future treatment.

If there is no history of prior psychiatric disturbance, it is important to rule out any physiological abnormalities that could produce these psychiatric symptoms. Many of the physiological changes that produce symptoms of delirium (confusion, disorientation, clouded consciousness) and dementia can also produce a variety of psychotic and psychological syndromes. If psychiatric symptoms are present, consideration should be given to a medical work-up similar to that for dementia or delirium. In addition, it should be kept in mind that a variety of non-Parkinsonian medications can produce these psychiatric symptoms, including antianxiety agents (e.g., diazepam, chloradiazepoxide), antihypertensive agents, steroids, antiulcer agents (e.g., cimetidine), as well as antidepressant and antipsychotic medications. Hence, part of the evaluation of any psychiatric symptoms should be a careful review for other superimposed medical disorders and medications that may bring about the psychiatric symptoms noted.

If medication effects and/or interactions and other medical problems are ruled out, it is appropriate to consider the best means of managing these symptoms. Behavioral management, environmental restructuring, and supportive psychotherapy can be quite effective in managing these symptoms. However, if psychiatric symptoms are unresponsive to behavioral and/or psychotherapeutic interventions, drug therapies are appropriate and should be prudently utilized.

In general, the choice of medications is related to the nature of the psychiatric symptoms as well as the status of the underlying Parkinson's disease. Initially, it may be most appropriate to consider a reduction of anti-Parkinsonian agents if possible. A reduction of anticholinergic medication may ameliorate symptoms of dementia or delirium, while reductions in dopaminergic medications may be effective for diminishing or extinguishing sleep disturbances, acute psychotic behavior with auditory hallucinations and delusions, as well as associated paranoia. In general, if a patient has a prior history of schizophrenia, it may be preferable to use anticholinergic agents in treating the Parkinson's disease since dopaminergic agents can likely exacerbate the underlying schizophrenia.

If the use of antipsychotic agents is deemed appropriate, medications such as chlorpromazine or thioridazine—both of which have more anticholinergic properties—may be less likely to exacerbate the Parkinson's disease. However, these same agents may be more likely to produce postural hypotension (a drop in blood pressure when rising to one's feet, which may produce dizziness and result in falls) and to produce signs and symptoms of anticholinergic toxicity and delirium. Dosages may need to be carefully measured and use limited to the shortest duration necessary to manage the symptoms. As noted above, antidepressant medication can also be usefully employed when depressive symptoms are more consistent and prominent in the clinical picture. Again, the more anticholinergic agents, such as imipramine or doxepin, may be better for Parkinson's disease, but they can produce side effects similar to antipsychotic medications. Antidepressants with lower anticholinergic potential (e.g., desipramine, maprotilene, and trazodone—which are also less sedating) may be more desirable.

Benzodiazepines and antianxiety agents can also be useful for symptoms related to anxiety and sleep difficulties. If deemed appropriate, agents with shorter half-lifes and no active metabolites (e.g., lorazapam, oxazepam, and alprazolam) are often preferable to benzodiazepines with longer half-lifes and active metabolites (e.g., diazepam, chloradiazepoxide, clorazepate) in patients who are older. In general the use of barbiturates (e.g., phenobarbital, secobarbital, amobarbital) should be avoided; they tend to produce paradoxical agitation, to suppress the relaxing REM (rapid eye movement) sleep, and cause adverse drug interactions. Antihistamines (e.g., diphenhydramine) can be useful as sleeping agents but are also more likely to cause confusion and delirium and to exacerbate dementia because of their anticholinergic properties. Likewise, chloral hydrate can be useful as a sleeping agent, but it, too, has the potential for interacting with other medications that older patients may be taking (e.g., anticoagulants such as warfarin). Hence, these considerations should be borne in mind when considering drug therapies for anxiety or sleep problems.

CONCLUSION

In conclusion, psychiatric symptoms and disorders occur with sufficient frequency in Parkinsonian patients to warrant familarity with their manifestations and the factors that help to produce them. An awareness of how psychiatric problems present themselves and how each member of the health care team can contribute to more effective management of these problems can be useful to anyone involved in the treatment of patients with Parkinson's disease.

BIBLIOGRAPHY

Celesia, G., and Wanamaker, W. "Psychiatric Disturbances in Parkinson's Disease." *Diseases of the Nervous System* 33 (1972): 577–583.

Cummings, J., and Benson, D. F. "Subcortical Dementia: Review of an Emerging Concept." *Archives of Neurology* 41 (1984): 874–879.

DeSmet, Y.; Ruberg, M.; Serdaru, M.; Dubois, B.; Lhermitte, F.; and Agid, Y. "Confusion, Dementia, and Anticholinergics in Parkinson's Disease." *Journal of Neurology, Neurosurgery and Psychiatry* 48 (1982): 1161–1164.

Duvoisin, R. *Parkinson's Disease: A Guide for Patient and Family,* 2d ed. New York: Raven Press, 1984.

Fonda, D. "Parkinson's Disease in the Elderly: Psychiatric Manifestations." *Geriatrics* 40 (1985): 109–114.

Harvey, N. "Psychiatric Disorders in Parkinsonism." *Psychosomatics* 27 (1986): 91–103 (pt. 1) and 175–184 (pt. 2).

Klawans, H. "Levodopa-Induced Psychosis." *Psychiatric Annals* 8 (1978): 447–451.

Lees, A., and Smith, E. "Cognitive Deficits in the Early Stages of Parkinson's Disease." *Brain* 106 (1983): 257–270.

Mindham, R. "Psychiatric Symptoms in Parkinsonism." *Journal of Neurology, Neurosurgery and Psychiatry* 33 (1970): 188–191.

Schwab, R.; Fabing, H.; and Prichard, J. "Psychiatric Symptoms and Syndromes in Parkinson's Disease." *American Journal of Psychiatry* 107 (1951): 901-907.

Thompson, T.; Moran, M.; and Nies, A. "Psychotropic Drug Use in the Elderly." *New England Journal of Medicine* 308 (1983): 134–138 (pt. 1) and 194–199 (pt. 2).

10

Coping with Depression

Raye Lynne Dippel

As many as half of all Parkinsonian patients suffer from depression, compared to only 10 percent of the general population. Although the depression that Parkinsonian patients suffer is typically mild, a significant number report moderate to severe depression.

Some investigators have argued that the depression suffered by Parkinsonian patients is a reaction to the chronic impairment in motor functioning; that is, depression is secondary to the discomfort and inconvenience of the disease. However, several studies have found Parkinsonian patients to be significantly more depressed than other groups of patients who suffer from the chronic and irreversible motor impairment such as that brought on by arthritis. Also, there does not appear to be a relationship between the severity of the depression and the duration or severity of Parkinson's disease, which runs counter to the hypothesis that the depression is primarily a reaction to the debilitating effect of the disease.

The increased prevalence of depression in Parkinsonian patients is most likely a result of reduced levels of brain monoamines, also called neurotransmitters. Neurotransmitters are the chemicals that allow nerve cells in the brain to communicate with one another and to send signals to muscles or sensory organs. Neurotransmitters are also important in the regulation of moods. The four major kinds of neurotransmitters include dopamine, norepinephrine, serotonin, and acetylcholine. Parkinson's disease is associated with a depletion of dopamine (see chapter 1). Norepinephrine and serotonin are also somewhat depleted in the brains of Parkinson's victims, and these monoamines are also known to be depleted in the brains of depressed individuals. In fact, antidepressant medication acts to increase brain monoamines.

There are many other factors that may contribute to the development of depression. Many individuals with Parkinson's disease are greatly frustrated by the rigidity, akinesia, and the tremor that interferes with their ability to complete even the most simple task, whether it be buttoning a shirt or writing a check. When the ability to move from place to place is made difficult, individuals may restrict their social activity, thereby intensifying feelings of loneliness and isolation. Parkinsonian patients report embarrassment at their tremor, their shuffling gait, and their poor posture. A friend of mine who has the disease disclosed that he no longer goes to church because people stare at him.

The frustration that Parkinsonian patients feel may express itself as the appearance of being irritable, demanding, or excessively dependent. These behaviors put stress on marital and family relationships. The guilt associated with placing extra burdens on family members tends to lower the patients' self-esteem. If the patients' activities are severely restricted, they may necessitate early retirement along with its accompanying financial worries. New activities must be developed to prevent the onset of boredom. The fear experienced when contemplating an unknown future or personal mortality must be faced head on. Given that Parkinsonian patients may have a biological propensity toward the development of depression, besides the stressors just discussed, it is very important that the physician, the nurse, the psychologist, or a family member recognize signs of depression and act to treat the disorder.

DIAGNOSIS OF DEPRESSION

Depression may not be readily apparent. Elderly depressed patients often do not present the same complaints witnessed in depressed younger adults. Elderly patients may not describe themselves as depressed, preferring instead to suffer quietly in a strong, stoic manner, perhaps fearful of being even more of a burden to their families. The depressed elderly may be less likely than younger persons to discuss openly feelings of despair, poor self-esteem, and worthlessness; older persons may be less inclined to complain of guilt.

The elderly are more likely to complain about feeling tired, loss of energy, sleeplessness, poor appetite, or a vague array of physical problems. It is often difficult to determine if these complaints are solely due to the Parkinsonism, or if depression has intensified their severity. The depressed elderly are less prone to tears than are younger depressed patients, and may be more likely to expess their depression by appearing irritable, on edge, or quick to anger. Those elderly who are suffering from depression frequently complain of memory problems or mental confusion.

It is important to identify depressed Parkinsonian patients and to treat the depression quickly and completely. Depression can be a fatal disorder: the risk of suicide in the elderly is many times greater than for younger people experiencing depression, and it may be four times greater for a depressed male than for a depressed female. Widowed and divorced individuals are also at considerable risk. Parkinsonian patients are at greater risk than most groups: the presence of a physical illness greatly increases the likelihood of suicide in the elderly. These losses are a real tragedy, because depression is an illness that can be treated with good results in most cases.

If a Parkinsonian patient discusses thoughts of suicide, take these statements seriously. Don't fall victim to the popular myth that if an individual talks about suicide, then he will be less likely to follow through. In most cases the victim does make an effort to let others know how much pain he is experiencing. Empathizing with those who suffer depression, taking their suicidal threats seriously, and acting immediately to find suitable treatment will go a long way toward saving lives.

Although Parkinsonian patients may run a greater risk of depression, occasionally the caregiver may also fall victim to depression. The increased stress of a changed lifestyle, resentment about assuming added responsibilities, and the guilt fostered by resentment toward the increased dependency of a loved one, may at times be more than caregivers can bear by themselves. Fear of hurting a spouse or family member often leads to silent suffering, and ultimately to depression. If this occurs, it is important that the caregiver receive treatment.

TREATMENT FOR DEPRESSION

Traditional methods of treating depression are recommended for Parkinsonian patients: antidepressants have generally been found to diminish the symptoms (see chapter 9). The combined treatment of levodopa and antidepressants is generally well tolerated by Parkinsonian patients. These antidepressants are often started at low dosages and increased slowly. As with most medication prescribed for the elderly, lower dosages may be used than for younger adults and serious consideration must be given to the effects of combining various drugs. Monoamine oxidase inhibitors, another type of antidepressant, are not considered safe when taken in conjunction with levodopa. Electroconvulsive therapy (shock treatment) is sometimes useful in treating severe cases of depression that do not respond to other forms of therapy.

In addition to drug therapy, depressed Parkinsonian patients may need counseling. Mental health assistance may aid victims of Parkinson's disease in their efforts at adjusting to this progressively debilitating illness; it is particularly important when the patient is also suffering from depression.

Let me stress that severely disturbed behavior need not be present for counseling to be either warranted or helpful. Clinical psychologists and other mental health professionals are trained to help patients and caregivers discuss openly fears and feelings that may be difficult to share with others.

STRATEGIES TO COMBAT DEPRESSION

Many things can be done to prevent feelings of depression or to diminish such debilitating feelings if they occur. When depression sets in, simple tasks and activities become difficult if not insurmountable. To combat these obstacles, start with small goals and gradually increase expectations in a slow, progressive manner. Do not invite failure by setting goals that cannot be reached. Parkinsonian patients should be very specific in describing their goals; effective means should be provided to evaluate whether these goals have actually been accomplished. If stated goals have not been accomplished, patients should review the reasons for this and, if need be, modify their goals or develop new strategies for obtaining them. Everyone needs goals for their growth and development. When depression emerges, it is especially important to identify goals if feelings of helplessness and hopelessness are to be overcome.

POSSIBLE GOALS

* Meet a new friend this month.

* Exercise twenty minutes, three times a week.

* Read a new book in an unfamiliar subject area this week.

* Practice listening to someone's concerns and then ask for feedback regarding listening effectiveness.

* Organize and label photos by the end of the month.

* Call an old friend.

* Dictate stories of your own childhood so that your children (and possibly their children) can gain a sense of family history.

* Write a poem

Notice that well-formed goals often include a time frame for completion. We sometimes work better with deadlines, and these also provide specific time to review accomplishments and to reevaluate progress toward emotional and physical health. Patients might consider establishing the following ritual: every Sunday morning (or at some other established time) weekly goals are determined and those of the past week are evaluated. What a special way to share one's self with family or friends.

When Parkinsonian patients establish their goals, the following considerations are recommended:

1. Make goals realistically obtainable. Set small goals.

2. They should feel good about themselves when a goal has been successfully accomplished; an appropriate reward could be enjoyed.

3. When goals are not accomplished, develop new strategies or alter the goals to make them more attainable.

4. Do not belittle or trivialize goals or successes. Do not exaggerate failures!

5. Be expressive and creative in developing goals! Patients should consider doing things they have never done before. Be daring and playful!

To fight depression and promote good self-esteem and life satisfaction, goals should address the following areas:

Exercise

* walking

* stretching

* posture exercises

* speech exercises

* (if necessary) passive exercises like isometrics

* swimming

Structural Activities

* crafts

* gardening

* volunteer work

* reading

* writing

* movies

Social Interaction

* church

* volunteer work

* out-of-town visits

* entertaining

* shopping or lunching with a friend

* support group meetings

Improved Communication (with spouse, family, and friends)
Discuss the following feelings:

* fear

* loneliness

* embarrassment

* anger

* frustration

* hope(lessness)

* helplessness

* joy

* love

(Write or dictate letters that examine feelings and relationships. There is no need to mail them.)

REWARDS

Many people are stingy when it comes to rewarding themselves for their hard work and effort. Depressed individuals frequently feel they do not deserve rewards. These people need to find ways to feel special and important. The reward need not be elaborate or expensive: treating oneself to a shopping trip, a meal at a new restaurant, or just buying some flowers to brighten a room; calling a special friend or visiting a relative; enjoying a bubble bath or a relaxing day at the park. It is vital that Parkinsonian patients realize that they have value as human beings and they deserve all the good things in life.

NEGATIVE SELF-TALK

It is also important for patients to reduce self-critical statements such as "I'm no good to anybody," "I can't do anything," "I'm too slow, " etc. Caregivers may find it useful to count every negative self-statement and display the tally in a conspicious place. Patients will be surprised at how often they focus on what they cannot do rather than what they can do! Instead of focusing on failures, patients should review their positive accomplishments. Individuals should attempt to be as generous with self-evaluation as they are when assessing the accomplishments of others. For example, a patient might review his life and make the following list:

* I raised two wonderful children.

* I was a solid, dependable employee.

* I have a loving relationship with my spouse.

* I walked around the block today.

* I finished my library book.

* I helped my wife/husband (fill in with a special task) today.

If the patient is unable to determine positive accomplishments, then the depression may be well entrenched; a mental health professional may need to be consulted.

WHAT IS A CLINICAL PSYCHOLOGIST?

Clinical psychologists have an undeserved reputation for being the mental health professionals to whom "crazy" people go for help. Actually, the vast majority of work performed by psychologists focuses on quite ordinary individuals who find themselves confronting special problems in their lives. Generally, counseling is brief in duration and much less expensive than commonly believed.

There is often confusion regarding the distinction between different types of mental health practitioners. Psychiatrists, for example, have earned a medical degree and have completed a residency program in psychiatry. They provide counseling and are licensed to prescribe medication.

Psychologists have completed a doctoral program (Ph.D., Psy.D., or Ed.D.), which typically includes three to four years of course work and practical experiences, and a year of clinical internship. Before being licensed to practice independently, the psychologist must hold a doctoral degree, have one or more years of postdoctoral experience under the supervison of a licensed psychologist, and pass a state-administered examination. In most cases, individuals with master's degrees in psychology are referred to as psychological associates and must practice under the supervision of a licensed psychologist.

WHAT PSYCHOLOGISTS DO

Psychologists offer a wide variety of services to the public. Only a few of the available services will be discussed here.

Psychological Testing

One of the most valuable skills that a psychologist develops in training is the administration and interpretation of psychological tests. There are many kinds of tests, but some of the most commonly used are those designed to measure intelligence, personality variables, and neuropsychological functioning.

Intelligence testing and neuropsychological testing are often requested to assess possible brain impairment. Neuropsychological testing assesses the patient's cognitive functioning. These tests measure an individual's ability to remember, to calculate, to use language, and to think abstractly. Such testing is particularly important if there is some question of brain impairments due to stroke or to a neurological disorder such as Alzheimer's disease. Some Parkinsonian patients also suffer from cognitive impairment. If there is reason to suspect that the patient is showing cognitive decline, it is often helpful to undergo neuropsychological testing to measure areas of weakness and strength. The results of such testing may suggest adjustments that the family should make to ensure the patient's safety and to protect the patient from unreasonable expectations or demands.

It is often difficult to determine if mental confusion and forgetfulness are due to brain impairment or depression, since many depressed individuals complain of difficulty with memory and concentration. Neuropsychological testing and personality testing may be useful in locating the problem and indicating what form of treatment will be most appropriate.

A psychologist conducts personality testing to gather information regarding a patient's current emotional state and the personality variables that influence behavior. Personality assessment is particularly useful in diagnosing depression and in assessing the risks of suicide. It is also useful for suggesting what factors might be modified to enhance life satisfaction. Common personality tests include:

1. *Minnesota Multiphasic Personality Inventory (MMPI)*. This is a pencil and paper test with over four hundred questions regarding likes and dislikes, past and present emotional experiences, and physical symptoms.

2. *Rorschach Inkblot Test*. This famous projective test has no right or wrong answers. The subject "projects" internal experiences onto a neutral stimulus (the inkblot). This is a very useful tool for understanding how an individual perceives the world.

3. *Thematic Apperception Test (TAT)*. This is another projective test in which subjects are asked to tell a story suggested by several drawings.

4. *Depression Inventories*. These are composed of several question-naires specifically designed to assess depression.

INDIVIDUAL PSYCHOTHERAPY

Therapists differ as to style and approach toward treatment, and each client presents different issues and needs. Based on test results or an initial interview, individual therapy may be recommended to help clients work through issues that may be creating stress, dissatisfaction with life, or depression.

Therapy may be very brief, lasting one to eight sessions, or it may last for several years, depending on the client's needs. The average length of therapy is probably between six and twelve months. The expected duration of therapy should be discussed with the psychologist during the first couple of sessions. Problem-solving sessions may prove adequate when seeking solutions to obvious situational obstacles (e.g., loss of income, or lack of interesting daily activities). Alternatively, the therapist and the client may agree that the therapy sessions should focus on internal experiences, such as feelings of poor self-esteem and guilt.

Psychotherapy is a very personal process that relies heavily on a strong relationship between therapist and client. Trust is essential to a positive outcome. If for some reason the match does not "feel" right, and the client is dissatisfied with the therapist, these concerns should be addressed at the next session. If the client's dissatisfaction continues, another therapist may be the solution. The best security against an unsatisfactory experience is to seek counseling from individuals who have had extensive training and experience, and who have the proper credentials. Clients have every right to verify the credentials of prospective counselors.

MARITAL THERAPY

Occasionally, the best arena to tackle the client's problems is in the presence of the entire family, or in the presence of the spouse. If the husband and wife are having difficulty communicating their experiences or feelings to one another, or find that they argue constantly, a therapist may be able to intervene gently in such a way that a clearer understanding of issues is possible (see chapter 12).

When an individual develops Parkinson's disease, the entire family system changes: Husbands and wives who have always gotten along well together may suddenly find themselves arguing or, perhaps worse, not talking to one another. Real issues may be masked by arguments over inconsequential matters. Through therapy, the family may begin to explore their fears regarding changes in roles, increased dependencies, fears of losing a family member, as well as anger over having to assume extra responsibilities or over an inability to follow through with a responsibility that had been diligently carried out for years. Once the real issues are identified, constructive work can be done to improve the relationship and to confront the fears.

FAMILY THERAPY

Parkinson's disease generally afflicts individuals who are older. Aging spouses or family members may also have health concerns that inhibit their ability to care for the Parkinsonian patient. Increased demands may be placed on the patient's children or members of the extended family. Many sons and daughters will want to help as much as possible, but demands of work and their own young families may limit the resources and the time they can devote to their loved one who suffers with Parkinson's disease. Family therapy can be a valuable forum for reviewing the family's problems and needs, discussing possible solutions, and clarifying the expectations of each family member. Better communication will help prevent the resentment that pulls many families apart in times of stress.

CONCLUSION

If professional counseling is sought, a physician may be able to suggest a well-respected mental health practitioner. The psychology department of the nearest medical school, university, or major hospital may be able to recommend psychologists in the immediate vicinity who have received specialized training in aging. These specialists are referred to as geropsychologists.

Most health or medical insurance policies provide reimbursement for mental health services, but a careful inquiry to an insurance agent will clarify the services, restrictions, or limitations imposed by the carrier. Medicare allows reimbursement for psychological services, but with certain restrictions. Medicaid coverage of psychological services is typically more generous.

An interdisciplinary team approach to the treatment of Parkinson's disease can prove helpful. Each discipline has unique viewpoints and specialized skills, which together can focus on the whole person.

SUGGESTED READINGS

Chafetz, P. K. "Clinical Geropsychologists in Long-term Care Facilities." *Long-term Care Currents* 9 (1 Ross Laboratories, Columbus, Ohio, 1986).

Dye., C. J. "Psychologists' Role in the Provision of Mental Health Care for the Elderly." *Professional Psychology* 9 (1978): 38–49.

Fonda, D. "Parkinson's Disease in the Elderly: Psychiatric Manifestations." *Geriatrics* 40 (1985): 109–114.

11

Cognitive Change

Jeffrey W. Elias and J. Thomas Hutton

"Cognition" refers to the process by which individuals perceive, reason, think abstractly, remember recent and past events, as well as keep track of personal actions or thoughts. A discussion of this topic with respect to Parkinson's disease must include a consideration of expected "normal" age changes in cognition; that is, any changes in cognition related to the disease have to be evaluated against the normal aging process. The idea that aging might bring with it some potential loss of cognitive capacity makes us all rather nervous, even though "normal" aging results in only slight changes in cognitive ability.

Parkinson's disease is not typically thought of as a disease that results in a major loss of cognitive abilities. It is true that some percentage of individuals who have the disease will progress to a point of cognitive change similar to that observed with Alzheimer's disease. Unlike Alzheimer's, however, Parkinson's disease does not inevitably result in a major loss of cognitive function. Many of the cognitive changes that do occur may be barely noticeable beyond what would be expected during normal aging, changes that can be easily overcome. It is not known why cognitive loss occurs in some Parkinsonian patients and not others. This is one of the major puzzles for those who study cognition and Parkinson's disease.

SUBCORTICAL FUNCTIONING AND
CONTROL OF MOTOR MOVEMENT

The outer layer of the brain, the cortex, is the area most closely associated with thinking and the storage of memories. Unlike Alzheimer's disease, which is caused by destruction of nerve cells within the cortex, Parkinson's disease arises from the loss of nerve cells in brain areas below the cortex, in what is called the subcortical region. The disease affects the basal ganglia, an area of the brain that controls motor function (movement). As shown in figure 1 (p. 134), the basal ganglia actually consist of a number of subcortical (below the cortex) structures that, although not adjacent to one another, are considered a system. Since the motor symptoms of Parkinson's seem to be related primarily to changes that occur below the cortex level, this makes any cognitive changes that occur during the disease quite interesting, because one normally associates changes in cognitive functioning with changes at the cortical level, not the subcortical level. As a result, many of the cognitive changes that take place in Parkinsonian patients are quite subtle. Cognitive changes in patients with Parkinson's disease may also result from changes in the cortex.

For those who would like to do more advanced reading beyond this text, some definitions of terms will be provided here. The basal ganglia consists of the *striatum, pallidum, substantia nigra,* and the *subthalamic nucleus.* It is the lack of the dark pigmented cells in the substantia nigra area that characterizes Parkinson's disease. The cells in this area of the brain provide dopamine to the striatum (see figure 2, p. 135).

Conventional wisdom suggests that the symptoms of Parkinsonism begin at the point where there is a loss of 80 percent of the cells in the substantia nigra, resulting in a proportional loss of the dopamine content in the striatum. Because it is the cells providing the dopamine that are damaged, rather than the cells in the striatum that receive the dopamine, the substance can be replaced via drug therapy. In Huntington's disease, another well-known disorder involving the basal ganglia, the nigrostriatal pathway is intact, but the cells that receive the dopamine in the striatum are damaged. Thus, introducing dopamine via drug therapy is not helpful in Huntington's disease.

As the cells of the nigrostriatal area age their pigment becomes darker due to the accumulation of *neuromelanin,* which is considered a waste product derived from processing dopamine. With age the more heavily pigmented cells die first, leading many researchers to believe that the increased pigmentation of the cells renders them more vulnerable to damage

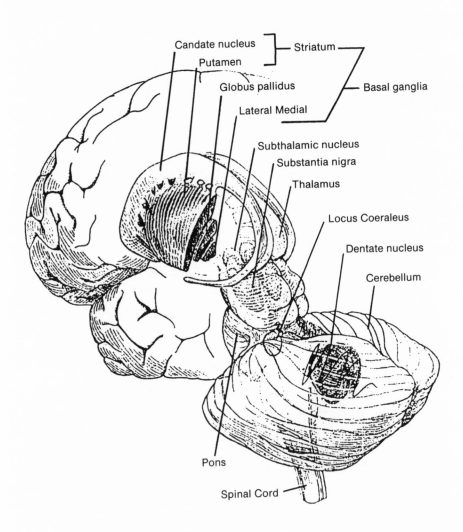

Figure 1.

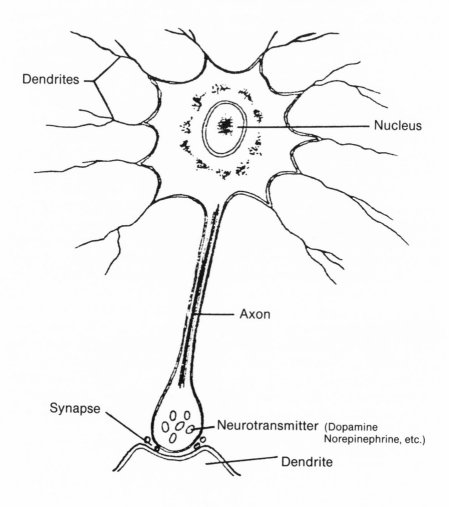

Figure 2.

from infectious agents or toxins. An example of this can be seen with animals that have been injected with the toxin MPTP, which has a particular affinity for the neuromelanin pigmented cells in the substantia nigra; the older the cells the more vulnerable they are to the toxin. With the normal aging process, one would expect a loss of the cells in the nigrostriatal area. In most individuals this loss is not thought to reach the 80 percent level—the suggested threshold for the onset of Parkinsonian symptoms. Given this relationship between cell loss in the nigrostriatal area and normal aging, however, it is not difficult to understand why it is often suggested that the changes in functioning—cognitive or motor—observed in Parkinson's disease represent an accelerated aging process.

SUBCORTICAL FUNCTIONING AND COGNITIVE CHANGE

Any discussion of the motor involvement noted in Parkinson's disease typically focuses on changes in the cell structure of the basal ganglia, as was just described. When the topic of *cognitive change* associated with Parkinsonism is raised, two other subcortical areas of the brain must be considered in addition to the basal ganglia. As shown in figure 3 (p. 137), these areas are the *locus coeruleus* and the *nucleus basalis of Meynert*. If we were trying to locate the locus coeruleus in the brain, we would find it covered by the cerebellum near the back of the brain, and located in the brainstem. (In textbooks, it is referred to as the upper pons area.) This is close to where the substantia nigra (the black pigmented area of the basal ganglia system that loses its dopaminergic neurons) is located. The locus coeruleus also contains the pigment neuromelanin, but the neuro-transmitter substance in this area of the brain is not dopamine but *norepine-phrine*. At norepinephrine nerve terminals an additional enzyme reaction converts dopamine to norepinephrine. Owing to the similar biochemical makeup of dopamine and norepinephrine, both are often referred to in the technical literature as monoamines or catecholamines. The major fiber tracts from the locus coeruleus make connections with the hypothalamus, the hippocampus, the cortex, the cerebellum, and the spinal cord. Similar to the normal aging process that takes place in the substantia nigra, the locus coeruleus also shows a normal age-related cell loss. The locus coeruleus and the nigrostriatal are two areas in the brain most likely to show a normal age-related loss of cells outside of any loss that might be associated with a disease such as Parkinsonism.

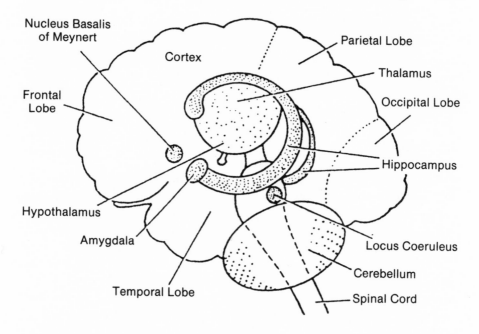

Figure 3.

The exact manner in which a partial loss of cells in the locus coeruleus will affect cognitive functioning is a matter of speculation. Experiments with animals have shown that destruction of this area of the brain by electrical lesions or toxins results in impaired learning and memory performance, and decreased attention and response to reward. Disease processes, however, do not typically result in the destruction of the area, and any effect of loss of cells in the locus coeruleus is probably a threshold effect; that is, a loss of cells up to a certain point can be withstood before any behavioral effects are observed.

A matter of increasing interest is the potential role of the locus coeruleus in determining sleep patterns. With age, sleep patterns change and less time is spent at certain stages of sleep, with increased awakenings. This erratic sleep pattern becomes more frequent in disease processes such as Parkinsonism where there is a loss of cells beyond the level expected during the normal aging process. As was pointed out in chapter 8, Parkinsonian patients frequently complain of sleep disturbance.

The third subcortical area linked to cognitive impairment in Parkinsonism is the *nucleus basalis of Meynert,* which is distinguished as a nucleus of cholinergic cells; that is, cells with acetylcholine as the neurotransmitter. Anatomy texts locate the nucleus basalis of Meynert by first locating the *basal forebrain neurons,* or the *substantia innominata.* The nucleus basalis of Meynert (as shown in figure 3) is one of the major groups of large cells found at the base of the forebrain. The nucleus basalis has links to the hippocampus and the entire cortex; it is a major source of cholinergic innervation of the cerebral cortex.

LABORATORY TESTS AND COGNITIVE FUNCTIONING

Given the above description of physiological changes to be expected with Parkinsonism, it should not come as a surprise that some cognitive change is expected beyond that observed with normal aging. As stated previously, not everyone with Parkinson's disease will show such changes, and it is not necessarily the case that such changes will critically interfere with functional capabilities. Some scientists have proposed that there may be different types of Parkinson's disease. In one type, changes occur in the brain similar to those seen with Alzheimer's disease, and dementia develops (see pp. 144-145). In the second type, the changes that occur in cognitive functioning are less severe.

To explore cognitive functioning in Parkinsonism (excluding dementia) a good overview can be had by examining: (1) general tests of intellectual functioning such as that provided by intelligence (IQ) tests, (2) studies focusing on memory, and (3) studies focusing on visual-spatial performance.

Intelligence Testing

A thorough review of research concerning intelligence test functioning in groups of Parkinsonian patients who do not suffer from dementia finds a mixed picture of outcomes. In some cases the groups show poorer performance overall than age-matched controls, and in some cases there is no difference at all. When there are differences between groups, it is usually only on some subtests of the intelligence tests and not all of the measures that make up an IQ test. In the studies of IQ tests we have completed in our own laboratory, we find a slight difference between Parkinsonians and age-matched controls that favors the latter. This is not a difference that could have any real functional importance. Repeated testing over a six-month period found little evidence of more rapid decline in intellectual functioning in the Parkinsonian group. In general, when there are differences between groups of Parkinsonian patients and control groups in intelligence test performance, these differences are not great and do not indicate any significant decline of intellectual processes in the Parkinsonian groups.

The most important finding of our research with intelligence tests is that shortened forms of these tests can be used reliably with Parkinsonian patients. We recommend their use because the longer versions of IQ tests are more tiring for patients and can negatively affect performance. In addition, we find that the use of generalized intelligence tests tells us very little about the changes in cognitive functioning that take place with Parkinsonism. IQ tests tap a range of abilities, and their use tells us that what we call intelligence is not greatly affected by Parkinsonism. The value of employing Parkinsonian patients as intelligence test subjects is that such examinations isolate unusual patterns of cognitive difficulty; i.e., patterns not normally associated with Parkinson's disease. An unusual pattern might indicate or identify other factors (e.g., tumor, stroke, depression, etc.) causing cognitive changes.

Memory

Memory is an easily observed and measured activity. It is not one process but many, and several types of memory can be measured. Though relatively easy to observe and measure, memory has to be carefully interpreted, most particularly because its performance is sensitive to a number of factors not related to age or disease. Researchers who use memory as a measure of cognitive performance know that there are normal fluctuations that everyone experiences. For example, knowing that one's memory is being tested can produce a level of stress strong enough to interfere with memory performance. Being comfortable with the test situation is as important for reducing interference as having prior experience of being tested.

There are several ways to approach the study of memory. The two most popular ways of organizing information are according to (1) the length of time information will be stored and (2) the kinds of information to be recalled.

Generally speaking, memory consists of two major components: *declarative* memory (facts and events) and *procedural* memory *(procedures and sequences)*. Many kinds of motor behaviors such as riding a bicycle or hitting a golf ball are thought to be procedural in nature. Often procedural memories are difficult to explain to someone else. (Try to explain to a friend how to learn to read efficiently when the material is upside down or backwards. It can be done, and it is a procedure, but difficult to explain.)

Declarative memory can be divided into memory for events/episodes (episodic memory) and memory for knowledge. Memory for words used to describe an event or to name an object is referred to as semantic memory. When one remembers an episode, a time element is involved, and events are recalled in sequence. In remembering a fact or a word, one does not necessarily remember the context or time period where it was learned. The knowledge is just retained and retrieved at the appropriate time.

When we discuss declarative and procedural memory we conceptualize in terms of the type of information stored. Memory can also be considered in terms of stages of processing. Within this model, information flows from one stage to the next in a sequence: *sensory, short-term* (divided into primary and secondary), and *tertiary* memory.

Sensory memory is thought to encompass the shear physical aspects of information. If one sees a word on a page or hears a word spoken, the initial representation of it is stored in sensory memory. Information must then be passed on to short-term storage where it is encoded (becomes meaningful in some way beyond being mere letters on a page or sound frequencies). How short is short-term memory? In the *primary* stage it can be very short indeed, perhaps only a few seconds or moments. Remembering a phone number or a name might be considered primary memory task. A common way to test primary memory in the laboratory is to provide a list of numbers, similar to a phone number, and ask a person to repeat the numbers very soon after hearing them. Most of us can remember about six or seven numbers before we start to have difficulty. If that name or phone number could be remembered for an hour, or a day, or maybe a week, but then forgotten, it would be said to be in the *secondary* portion of short-term memory. It is still short-term, but longer than primary.

One might reasonably ask at what point memory becomes long-term or *tertiary*, because it seems that what is designated as short-term, particularly secondary-short-term memory, is rather arbitrary. Indeed, it is arbitrary, and there is a lot of ground covered between what is considered primary memory and tertiary memory. Those memories that we seem to retain rather permanently can definitely be considered long-term. A process known as *consolidation* helps to make memories more permanent. Consolidation takes place over time and begins when information is first encountered at the sensory stage, and it continues through to the tertiary stage. It is suspected that even though memories are in long-term or tertiary (remote) memory, they may still be going through the process of consolidation.

The area of the brain where consolidation starts is the hippocampus, located in the cortex of the brain (see figure 3). (If you put your finger to the middle of your head just in front of the left or right ear, you would be pointing in the general direction of the hippocampus.) It is situated at a point where the cortex becomes very thin and rolls over on itself in single cell layers. When there is damage to this area of the brain it is most noticeable in terms of short-term memory loss; more specifically, secondary short-term memory loss. Primary memory remains intact even with extensive damage to the hippocampus. A blow to the head received in a traffic accident, let's say, may affect the functioning of the hippocampus. For example, amnesia is a form of short-term memory loss where new memories cannot be consolidated to a point where they are remembered for more than a few minutes.

Procedural memory does not seem to be as affected by damage to the hippocampus as is declarative memory. There have been cases where individuals with hippocampal damage (amnesia victims) have learned procedures as well as those without such damage, but have been unable to remember that they were trained, or unable to take advantage of repeated information or situations. It is primarily because of these kinds of findings that scientists consider procedural memory to be of a different kind than the memory for facts or events.

The kind of memory difficulty most likely to occur in normal aging is secondary or short-term memory processing. In Alzheimer's disease, which is the most common form of dementia, an inability to remember actions, events, or information for more than a few minutes is a primary symptom. Normal aging does not result in such drastic memory dysfunction: one is more likely to describe the memory dysfunction experienced in normal aging as forgetfulness.

We have all experienced short-term memory loss at one time or another. In many cases forgetfulness results from inattention, lack of interest, or lack of effort. Stress, fatigue, depression, preoccupation, or boredom can negatively affect consolidation at the level of secondary memory processing. Sometimes information is presented too quickly or simultaneously with competing information; this will interfere with memory consolidation as well. Both laypersons and professionals have to be very careful not to assume that forgetfulness in old age is a sign of impending dementia. Memory loss that occurs with normal aging is often referred to as *benign*. It may be annoying at times, but a person can still function quite well.

Sometimes depression can result in severe memory loss. When depression expresses itself in this form, it can be difficult to distinguish from more serious conditions such as Alzheimer's or stroke. Memory difficulty brought on by depression is usually selective; that is, there is no general or global loss of memories, but specific events and facts are lost. General organization abilities are still observable in memory, and often no attempt is made to make up information to cover the memory loss. With disease processes (e.g., Alzheimer's) organization abilities in general are affected, the loss is usually global in nature, and often attempts are made to cover up the loss.

Some researchers consider the memory changes that occur with Parkinsonism to represent an acceleration of the normal aging process. This concept is supported by the observation that memory difficulties associated with Parkinson's disease are most noticeable at the secondary memory processing and consolidation stages. The kinds of memory tasks that are likely to illustrate differences between Parkinsonian and control groups are those that require new material to be learned, organized, retained, and consolidated over more than a few minutes' time. A very good example would be the ability to remember the details of a short story over the time span of a few minutes. As a group, those with Parkinson's disease would be expected to remember fewer details of such a story, although the rate of forgetting over time might not differ between groups. Such a test of memory ability is also one of the most sensitive in detecting differences among age groups.

Research findings in our laboratory indicate that when considered as a group, Parkinsonian patients do not appear to take advantage of repeated information and may find it more difficult, when attempting to recognize old information, to discriminate items based on distinctive features that would help determine their familiarity. *Recognition memory* is the ability to recognize material or places as familiar, even if they cannot be specifically recalled. For example, when driving to work or to the store over familiar roads and streets, not only is the correct path being recalled, but it is being recognized as well. Sometimes, in more serious disease processes such as dementia, the directions to get to a place can be remembered, but the ability to recognize the surroundings is missing. This is a frightening experience, but in itself it does not constitute a diagnosis of some form of dementia. Extreme stress or tiredness can produce the same effect, as can drugs and medication, or physical illness. It is also not a symptom normally associated with Parkinson's disease. Typically, differences in recognition memory between those with Parkinsonism and control groups who are similar in age are very subtle and may only be detected with careful inspection in a laboratory.

One area of memory where we have found reliable differences related to Parkinson's disease is in the ability to remember visual-spatial patterns. Subjects have been asked to look at and remember line drawings of figures (e.g., squares, triangles, circles, etc.) for a few seconds. We then ask these subjects to recreate the figures a few seconds later. Not all, but many Parkinsonians experience difficulties with this task. Other investigators have reported the same findings, and this kind of difficulty with visual-spatial information processing and visual-spatial memory is thought to be a distinctive characteristic of Parkinsonism. At least one investigator has found that younger individuals who use the drug by-product MPTP, which damages the nigrostriatal tract (and as a result reduced the dopamine supply to the striatum), have visual-spatial memory difficulties. These individuals did not have the changes in the locus coeruleus and basal forebrain area typically associated with Parkinson's disease. Quite possibly the visual-spatial memory problems associated with Parkinsonism are related to the loss of dopamine. It is not clear how this might manifest itself functionally as patients try to navigate their environment. It should be noted that this is not the same kind of visual-spatial problem as not being able to recognize familiar surroundings. An area just beginning to gain attention in Parkinson's research relates changes in vision to changes in visual-spatial functioning. That is, rather than assume that all changes in visual-spatial processing are due to changes in higher-level functions in the brain, there is the suspicion that changes in the eye may contribute to poor visual-spatial performance.

With the exception of those who develop dementia, there is no evidence that Parkinsonism will severely affect the higher-order thinking and reasoning processes. In our research we find no evidence of cognitive slowing to accompany the motor slowing, which is a cardinal symptom of Parkinson's disease. Sometimes the repeating of some aspect of a task before going on to the next portion (perseveration) is seen more often in Parkinsonian patients than with normal aging. Generally speaking, the cognitive aspects of functioning are only weakly associated with the motor symptoms. Based on research in our own lab and the research of others, we have begun to gather evidence that persons who experience a later onset of Parkinson's disease, and who are older, will show (as a group) more difficulties with cognitive tasks than those who have had an earlier onset and perhaps longer duration of symptoms. This is particularly evident on visual-spatial tasks. We have also observed individuals who seem to have severe memory problems, yet they present a level of awareness and reasoning indicating that the memory loss is not a sign of dementia. We have observed only a few such individuals and, at this time, we are unable to determine what is contributing to the severe memory problem.

DEMENTIA AND PARKINSON'S DISEASE

The development of dementia is not considered a normal consequence of contracting Parkinson's disease, but the probability of developing dementia is higher in those with the disease. Estimating what percentage of Parkinsonians might be expected to develop a diagnosis of dementia is a difficult task. Estimates vary greatly in the literature. It is difficult to know what estimate to accept since the diagnosis of dementia in Parkinsonian patients has often not been done with the same care as in those cases where dementia is suspected as the primary diagnosis. Choosing only the largest studies and the ones using the most reliable criteria, we arrive at an estimate of 20 percent. It must be noted, however, that about 10 percent of those classified as demented in these studies were considered to have a fairly mild dementia. Furthermore, not very much is known about the progressive or global nature of dementia in Parkinson's disease. In Alzheimer's disease the decline is progressive and global in nature, eventually touching all aspects of cognitive functioning. The same kind of information is not available for Parkinsonism.

Dementia is a clinical-behavioral syndrome that needs to be carefully diagnosed to exclude treatable disorders such as depression, and to include definite functional disability and loss of orientation to time, place, and person. The prominent clinical signs of dementia include the global impairment of higher cortical functions affecting memory, judgment, initiation of action, social functioning, control of emotion, and the ability to carry out everyday tasks. While memory loss is often a cardinal symptom of dementia, it is neither a declaration of dementia nor the sole justification for a dementia diagnosis.

Overall it is estimated that there are potentially sixty disorders that can result in dementia syndromes. About 10 to 20 percent of these disorders are treatable and involve metabolic disorders, toxins, endocrine disorders, space occupying lesions, and psychiatric problems. If dementia is suspected, a neurologist should be consulted to determine if there is a need for additional medical treatment. By far the dominant physical condition leading to dementia is Alzheimer's disease. It is estimated that about 50 percent of those with dementia will have Alzheimer's disease, another 10 percent will have a combination of Alzheimer's disease and multi-infarct disease, and 10 percent will have multi-infarct disease without dementia. The remaining 30 percent can be attributed to other conditions. Typically, the diagnosis of dementia, particularly Alzheimer's disease, is in part one of exclusion. That is, many conditions need to be excluded before the diagnosis of Alzheimer's disease can be used.

It is not clear if the diagnosis of dementia that accompanies Parkinson's disease should be considered a separate type of dementia, or if it is actually Alzheimer's disease. The physical changes in the brain tissue of those diagnosed with Alzheimer's disease, such as neurofibrillary tangles, have also been found in the brain tissue of some Parkinsonian patients who have dementia. At this time, these physical manifestations of Alzheimer's disease are not thought to occur in all individuals with Parkinson's disease, only those of a particular subtype who develop dementia. Currently, there is no way of knowing which course Parkinson's disease will take: none of its clinical symptoms are predictive of dementia versus nondementia. While it has been suggested that the drugs used to treat the motor symptoms of Parkinsonism might be a cause of dementia, there is no evidence to support this notion. Occasionally, treatment with anticholinergics might result in a disturbance of short-term secondary memory, but these are temporary rather than long-term effects.

SUMMARY AND CHALLENGE FOR THE FUTURE

In addition to the motor symptoms and disabilities that are characteristic of Parkinson's disease, there may be changes in memory, visual-spatial orientation, and perception as well. Difficulties with short-term memory and the ability to recall visual-spatial material are the most prevalent cognitive changes. The degree, rate, and breadth of change in cognitive functioning accompanying Parkinsonism is at present impossible to predict. More information is needed to determine how such changes on neuropsychological tests relate to the overall ability to function in the home or office. In fact, the term "cognitive change" has been carefully chosen to reflect what is actually known to occur, rather than suggest the presence of a "cognitive deficit."

A small percentage of Parkinsonian patients will develop a dementia similar to that described as Alzheimer's disease. At this time there is no known set of symptoms or behaviors we can point to in the early stages of the disease that will indicate the eventual severity of the cognitive changes taking place. Suspicion that a severe change in cognitive function has taken place should be brought to the attention of health care professionals. In some cases, severe changes in cognition are the result of depression (see chapter 10) or other treatable medical disorders.

SUGGESTED READINGS

Chui, H. C.; Mortimer, J. A.; Slager, V.; Zarrow, C.; Bondareff, W.; and Webster, D. D. "Pathological Correlates of Dementia in Parkinson's Disease." *Archives of Neurology* 43 (1986): 991–95.

Elias, M. F.; Elias, J. W.; and Elias, P. K. "Biological and Health Influences on Aging." In J. E. Birren and K. W. Schaie (eds.) *Handbook of the Psychology of Aging.* New York: Academic Press, 1988.

Elias, M. F.; Elias, J. W.; and Elias, P. K. *Basic Processes in Adult Developmental Psychology.* St. Louis: Mosby, 1977.

Fisher, A.; Hanin, I.; and Lachman, C. *Alzheimer's and Parkinson's Disease: Strategies for Research and Development.* New York; Plenum Press, 1986.

Huber, S. J.; Shuttleworth, E. C.; and Paulson, G. W. "Dementia in Parkinson's Disease." *Archives of Neurology* 43 (1986): 987–90.

Mann, D. "The Locus of Coerulus and It's Possible Role in Ageing and Degenerative Disease of the Human Central Nervous System." *Mechanisms of Aging and Development* 23 (1983): 73–79.

Mann, D. M.; and Yates, P. O. "Pathogenesis of Parkinson's Disease." *Archives of Neurology* 39 (1982): 545–49.

Nauta, W.; and Freitag, M. *Fundamental Neuroanatomy,* New York: Freeman and Co., 1986.

Whitehouse, P. J.; Hedreen, J. C.; White, C. L.; and Price, D. L. "Basal Forebrain Neurons in the Dementia of Parkinson's Disease." *Annals of Neurology* 13 (1983): 243–48.

12

Parkinson's Disease and the Family

Karen Boyd Worley and Raye Lynne Dippel

When an individual suffers from Parkinson's disease, it is not just a personal matter but a reality that affects every member of the family. Parkinson's disease taxes the family's financial, physical, and emotional resources. The uncertainty and doubt prior to diagnosis, the hardship of new symptoms and setbacks, and for some the heartbreaking necessity of nursing home care combine to test a family's best coping skills. At times, family members rise above the difficulties and demonstrate not only adequate adjustment but also inspiring personal growth. On other occasions, the stress becomes too much and families begin to behave in dysfunctional ways.

All families are clearly challenged by the presence of Parkinson's disease in one of their members. What accounts for the ability of some families to struggle through hard times—to form uniquely workable solutions to their situation—while others seem to become mired in unpleasant, hurtful, or unhealthy interactions? Why do certain families find themselves able to cope well at some times and poorly at others? While there are no hard and fast answers to the complex and unique workings of an individual family, systems theory offers a way of looking at how families interact and offers suggestions to "helping" professionals in their efforts to facilitate a family's move beyond unpleasant or unhealthy situations.

SYSTEMS THEORY AND THE BIOMEDICAL APPROACH

The Parkinson's disease symptoms in which family influence may be particularly important are depression and cognitive impairment (see chapters 10 and 11). The beneficial effects of levopoda, so helpful for motor symptoms, are of no use in alleviating these two secondary complaints. Between 30 and 40 percent of all Parkinsonian patients have shown low levels of depression, but these are consistently higher than other comparison groups, healthy or ill. It is apparent in many cases that when an individual patient responds positively to levodopa, thus reducing physical symptoms and increasing ability to be active, depression decreases. In this situation, *hope* for maintaining gains may be as important as an increased activity level.

Considering the progressive nature of the disease, it is no wonder that a diagnosis of Parkinsonism can have a profound emotional effect on patients and their loved ones. This gives support to the notion that depression associated with the disease is not entirely physiologically based. The positive or negative adjustment of patients and their families to this situation is often closely related to the patients' level of depression. In addition, problems not necessarily related to Parkinson's disease at all—such as the loss of a spouse, family problems, financial difficulties, or other psychosocial stress—can contribute to depression.

The family may have an indirect impact on the patient's level of cognitive impairment. Between 20 and 30 percent of Parkinsonian patients have cognitive impairments serious enough to cause significant difficulty in their lives. Even more, perhaps the majority, report some decline in their mental capacities. But, like depression, there are other factors in a patient's life that may contribute to cognitive impairment. For example, typical symptoms of the mask-like face; soft, slurred speech; and difficulty maneuvering, all contribute to social isolation and apathy. Certainly, as patients become more isolated and apathetic, environmental stimulation is significantly diminished. This lack of stimulation contributes to the likelihood of depression and decreased intellectual stimulation, which in turn can cause an existing cognitive impairment to appear even more serious than it is.

It is important to caution families and professionals alike that the presence of depression or cognitive impairment does not automatically indicate a problem in the care that a particular family is giving or in the attitude with which the care is given. These are both common symptoms of the disease that do not respond to effective drug therapy. Depression does respond to other medications, which can be prescribed by a physician.

THE MYTH OF THE NORMAL FAMILY

The myth of the "normal" family suggests that such a family does not experience stress. With that definition, it would certainly be a challenge to find even one temporarily "normal" family. A typical fairy tale ending to a love story is "and so they got married and lived happily ever after." As anyone with a family knows, that is when the trouble just begins! Salvador Minuchin, a major contributor to the concept of structural family therapy, describes the myth of placid normality in a family without stress as just that—a myth. Certainly the presence of Parkinson's disease exacerbates whatever stress is present. By way of illustration, a man who has had an on-going conflict with his mother-in-law is not likely to have a miraculous new love and appreciation for her just because she has developed Parkinson's disease. Instead, the "normal" level of stress generated between mother-in-law and son-in-law may increase to disruptive proportions as involvement between the two families changes due to the disease.

APPLYING FAMILY SYSTEMS THERAPY

Family systems therapy can provide guidelines for evaluation and treatment intervention without necessarily creating a special category for the family that does its best to cope with a difficult situation. Systems "theory" is the result of the rather unremarkable observation that people are influenced by others and by the way they interact with one another.

Several key ideas in systems theory will be discussed in the context of families dealing with Parkinson's disease; these ideas will illustrate the potential usefulness of this approach. These systems theory ideas, suggested by Minuchin, include family as an entity:

1. having a *structure* that must constantly undergo transformation,
2. undergoing specific *stages* of development that require restructuring, and
3. needing to *adapt to changed circumstances* to maintain continuity and enhance the social growth of each member.

STRUCTURE

The structure of a family may be explained by defining subsystems, or functional groups of members. These subsystems may be formed according to age, function, sex, or other factors. For example, the spouse subsystem consists of the husband and wife. It serves as a refuge for the couple and is a source of authority in the family. The sibling subsystem gives a child an opportunity to learn skills in negotiating and competing with other children. Subsystems that cross generational boundaries may include a parent, a grandparent, and/or a child. In a well-functioning family the subsystems have clear but flexible boundaries. Parents have a strong alliance in which they support each other and do not allow the children to mediate problems that are appropriately handled by adults. Likewise, a healthy adult family does not allow the parents to mediate all problems.

When Parkinson's disease strikes a person at the top of the family hierarchy it can throw the whole family structure into disarray. In many families the adult children may rigidly cling to the familiar authority patterns: together with the ill parent, the children may conspire to deny the severity of symptoms in order to preserve the authority of the family patriarch or matriarch. In such a situation, appropriate care may not be provided. Some "role reversal" would be appropriate: the children may need to help care for the parent rather than the other way around. For example, an aged mother with Parkinson's disease may insist on continuing to cook a large Thanksgiving dinner for the entire family, despite the fact that she suffers from emotional stress and physical strain. Her children could offer to host the dinner or contribute to the cooking and cleaning. It is important, however, not to rob Parkinsonians of opportunities to assist and participate (albeit moderately) in all their usual activities. Responsibilites may shift but personal dignity must never be ignored.

Stages

Familial structure reveals a great deal about a family at a given point in time, but not necessarily how the family changes over time. According to a number of therapists and theorists, most families progress through predictable stages in their group life cycle. Each stage is initiated by a particular life event that requires change and adjustment by every family member. One of the family's basic tasks is to intergrate stability and change so that the unit, as well as each of its individual members, can grow without becoming stuck or overwhelmed by sudden, drastic changes. Each stage presents the family with specific tasks that must be mastered. The traditional stages that a family passes through are (1) courtship, (2) marriage and becoming a couple, (3) childbirth and young children, (4) middle marriage with school-age children, (5) late middle age when children begin leaving home, and (6) old age. There are typical problematic patterns indicating that the family is not handling the new changes. Poor resolution at any one stage makes resolution at later stages more difficult. The most common types of stage-related problems are (a) normal acute stage specific difficulties, (b) maladaptive responses to the specific pressures of a given stage, and (c) chronic problems related to unresolved issues from some prior developmental stage(s).

Members of the typical family may be at different stages, which further complicates family systems. For instance, a family consisting of a husband and wife may have several grown children in varying stages of leaving home, getting married, or having their own children. The parents of this couple may be in the stage of "old age" with complications that leave them more dependent on their children. This husband and wife family may not only have the responsibility of caring for their own children (and probably their grandchildren), but their parents as well.

Families who get "stuck" in one of these stages, may find it difficult to function effectively. In one family interviewed, John and Ellen* had four children. The youngest had learning disabilities that resulted in delayed emotional maturity (this twenty-five-year-old son was routinely unemployed and living at home). The other children had gone through divorces, and during the last seven years one or more of them had moved back into the home temporarily. In addition, John and Ellen had assumed important responsibilities for the daily care of their grandchildren. Clearly, this family was finding it difficult to move successfully through the stage of "children leaving home."

Both John and Ellen had major health complications of their own. (Ellen had recently undergone successful treatment for cancer.) Both John and Ellen worked full time. The family was obviously experiencing multiple stressors that John and Ellen were attempting to mediate. As might be expected, such stressors resulted in several levels of conflict: marital, parent-child, and sibling. In addition, Ellen's father, a widower, developed Parkinson's disease and mild dementia, which rendered him unable to care for himself. He had always lived near-by and depended on his daughter for

---

*These names are fictitious.

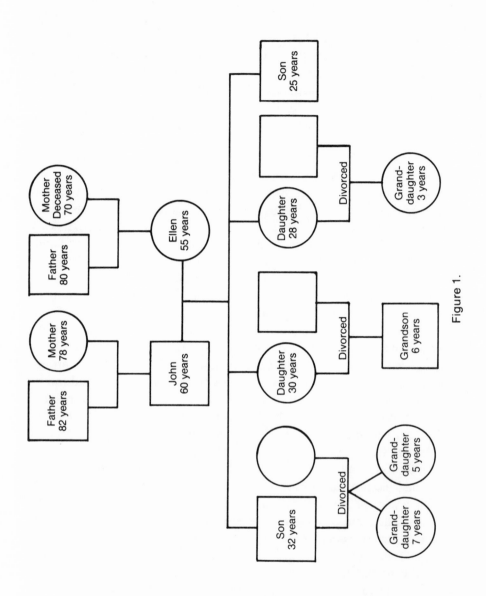

Figure 1.

assistance in managing his home. All family members "assumed" that Ellen would care for him.

Through trial and error, this family made adjustments that encouraged successful movement through the stage of "children leaving home," which resulted in less stress and greater independence for all family members. The children were encouraged to reside outside of the home, and the parents were more realistic about what they were capable of doing for their children. An apartment was built in the back of the house to allow Ellen's father more independence and privacy in a safe environment where he would benefit from frequent family interaction. This offered John and Ellen greater opportunities to have their "alone" times, during which they would go on frequent weekend trips, thereby reducing the stress brought on by family members always "asking" for assistance. The children had grown to be very dependent on their parents for help in a wide variety of ways, from unstopping the commode, to watching the grandchildren, to sewing a new dress, or making a loan, etc. With gentle encouragement, the children learned to rely on themselves or to find others in the community to assist them with their projects. Ellen's brother and sister were also invited to play a greater role in the care of their father. Although these adjustments were difficult to make, the family has generally resolved the stage of "children leaving home," and a much calmer, more loving family atmosphere exists.

Another family had been relatively successful during the "children leaving home" stage, that is until their mother developed Parkinson's disease. The adult children (now married) who were enjoying thriving relationships with their spouses and children, became very concerned and anxious about their mother's fragile appearance and her diminished ability to manage her own affairs. She had always been a fiercely independent, professional woman who managed on her own.

As the disease progressed, the family members came under increasing stress: Her oldest son, who lived several hundred miles away, began booking frequent trips home to arrange for his mother's care and to maintain the company she owned. These added duties put considerable stress on his marriage and limited the time he could spend with his young children. Conflicts soon arose between the adult children. For example, the older children were angered by the continued demands that their youngest brother made on their mother. His siblings had always resented the relatively few restrictions placed on their "baby" brother during his formative years: he typically eluded punishment for infraction of rules, and generally he got whatever he wanted. The youngest brother's current lack of sensitivity to his mother's needs and limitations infuriated the other children, who not only argued with him but found themselves confronting their mother, who defended him. These conflicts increased the family's stress levels and presented strong roadblocks to successful group problem solving and adjustment.

These are just a few examples of how the inherently complicated tasks of normal life stages can become even more difficult to accomplish when a family member has Parkinson's disease. In such situations, short-term family therapy with a mental health professional experienced in family counseling and familiar with the special problems of Parkinson's disease may be helpful. Such assistance may foster reorganization of resources and hasten movement though the tasks at hand. The following case history* illustrates how one couple coped with the diagnosis and development of the wife's Parkinson's disease as they entered the stage of retirement and old age.

Martha and George had been married for many years when Martha was diagnosed with Parkinson's disease. For several weeks she relied heavily on the support of her minister as she struggled to find the courage to tell her husband. Martha's fears were well founded. George was devastated by the news; he remembered the effect that Parkinson's disease had on a relative and her family at a time well before the advent of effective drug therapy. George saw his hopes for a comfortable retirement dashed. Of even greater importance were his concerns for Martha's well-being.

Somehow, George and Martha clung together as they tried to comfort one another in this time of overwhelming confusion. Now, years later, Martha is at a good level of adjustment in the course of her illness. She and George have worked out an "optimal" regimen of diet, exercise, social activity, and scheduling of medication, which allows Martha several hours of rewarding activity per day. The couple emphasizes "flexibility" as their most important policy in reducing stress. Although George is the identified caregiver in the relationship, he notes the tremendous emotional support he gets from his wife. He gratefully points out her strength and support when he suffered a heart attack a few years ago.

Adapting to Changed Circumstances

A family is subjected not only to inner pressure from developmental changes in its members and subsystems, but also from outer pressures that may

---

*The names have been changed.

result from problems one or more family members may have with work, school, church, the law, the economy, or any of a number of outside influences. Integral to the process of change and continuity that the family must accomplish are the stresses of accommodating new situations constantly presented by family members and the community. While all families must cope with these changes, more serious problems arise when families increase the rigidity of their relationship patterns and boundaries in response to stress and avoid or resist exploration of any alternatives.

An example of this is the case of Mary and Herbert* who had mutually agreed that Herbert was head of the household and breadwinner, while Mary was the homemaker and cook. Both had stringent expectations for an immaculate household and regular home-cooked meals. As Mary became progressively more disabled with Parkinson's disease, it became more difficult for her to live up to this standard. She voiced her complaints to friends and relatives, but not to her husband. Herbert did not recognize the need to take over some of the household responsibilities, despite his retirement and his wife's disability. More seriously, he did not understand how hurt and disappointed Mary was at her perception of his lack of support in her time of need. This stress exacerbated her symptoms. Both became more and more frustrated, irritable, and depressed, making it more difficult to bridge the widening gap between them. Herbert perceived his wife's increasing difficulty in performing everyday activities as malingering, which he resented. As communication became more tense and less productive, even simple solutions, such as hiring someone to help around the house or occasionally allowing family members to bring in food, could not lessen the resentment between Herbert and Mary. While early intervention by a mental health professional probably would not have changed their long-held beliefs about the roles they expect men and women to have in marriage, it might have allowed Herbert and Mary to come to grips with her illness, to communicate with one another directly when problems needed to be solved, and to recognize their need for each other's support in a time of difficult transition.

Rigid boundaries erected by husbands and wives sometimes cause them not to let any "outsiders" help. David and Elaine** kept David's illness a secret even from their grown children for a number of years after the initial diagnosis of Parkinson's disease. This effectively barred the children

---

*Names and identifying information have been changed.
**The names have been changed.

from providing help for their father and mother, both of whom had health problems. Elaine performed her duties so well that her husband became increasingly passive, dependent, and fragile. After Elaine's death, the children and a live-in companion allowed David to remain successfully in his own home. Despite grief over his wife's death, David has been able to take a stronger hand in directing his own medical care and daily activities. In this situaiton, it was Elaine's unfortunate death that was instrumental in loosening up boundaries that allowed help from family and a live-in companion to come in and for David to strengthen his contacts with the outside world. A sensitive recognition of Elaine's hovering care by a concerned health professional could have allowed encouragement of beneficial use of family members and community resources before her death, thus aiding this couple's adaptation to changing circumstances.

FAMILY INTERVENTION PRIORITIES

The list of questions in table 1 was developed by Remnet to assist families in examining their interactions and to assess their adjustment to a chronic disabling illness in a family member.

TABLE 1

FAMILY ASSESSMENT
(Remnet, 1979)

1. Is the family currently in crisis?

2. Has the family system changed to meet needs?

3. Is change acknowledged and accepted?

4. Who is assuming responsibility for what?

5. Is responsibility realistic?

6. Is the whole family involved in the plan?

7. Have family members' expectations been defined?

8. Is the current plan considered permanent or temporary?

Zarit and his colleagues suggest that good problem-solving skills are essential in making successful adjustments and adaptations to a chronic disease such as Parkinson's disease. The following guidelines (see table 2) adapted from his book might provide a framework from which to begin working on major family problems.

TABLE 2

PROBLEM-SOLVING PROCESS
(Zarit, Orr, and Zarit, 1985)

1. Identify the problem.
   a. antecedents
   b. consequences

2. Generate alternative solutions.
   (No censoring)

3. Select a solution: pros and cons.

4. Cognitive rehearsal of plan.

5. Carry out the plan.

6. Evaluate outcome.

CONCLUSION

A genuine systems perspective must recognize the reciprocal influences of the individual, the family, and other systems. The medical community is a primary system that families must face when one of their members is diagnosed as having Parkinson's disease. It is critical that the health care professional dealing with these families address the impact of the illness and the stress of caregiving with preexisting or current stresses in designing clinical care for families. Family-oriented professionals must appreciate what it means for families to have a member develop serious and long-term dysfunction, and how difficult it is for families to cope over time, especially when they shoulder the burden of primary caregiving. The medical community can respond to this need by seeing that appropriate mental health services are available. Services should include crisis intervention; brief, problem-focused family therapy; and multiple family groups. Additionally, mental health workers dealing with families of Parkinson's patients need specific data about the symptoms, progress, and treatment of the disease in order to provide the family with emotional support, information, and referral to needed resources such as support groups, home and respite care services, and nursing homes. The successful collaboration of physicians and mental health professionals can help Parkinsonian patients and their families in achieving optimal adjustment.

SUGGESTED READINGS

Dakof, G. A., and Mendelson, G. A. "Parkinson's Disease: The Psychological Aspects of a Chronic Illness." *Psychological Bulletin* 99 (1986): 375–87.

Grinspoon, L. (ed.) "Family Therarpy—Part I." In *The Harvard Medical School Mental Health Letter* 4 (1988): 1–4.

Karpel, M. and Strauss, E. "The Family Life Cycle." In *Family Evaluation.* New York: Gardner Press, Inc., 1983, pp. 49–77.

Minuchin, S. *Families and Family Therapy.* Cambridge, Mass.: Harvard University Press, 1977.

Montalvo, B., and Thompson, R. "Conflicts in the Caregiving Family." *The Family Therapy Networker.* (July/August 1988): 30–35.

Rodeheaver, D., and Datan, N. "The Challenge of Double Jeopardy: Toward a Mental Health Agenda for Aging Woman." *American Psychologist* 43 (1988): 648–54.

Walsh, F., and Anderson, C. "Chronic Disorders and Families: An Overview." *Journal of Psychotherapy and the Family* 3 (1987): 3–32.

Zarit, H.; Orr, N.; and Zarit, J. *The Hidden Victims of Alzheimer's Disease: Families Under Stress.* New York: New York University Press, 1985.

13

Community Support Systems

Susan Imke and J. Thomas Hutton

The purpose of this chapter is to suggest ways in which Parkinsonians and their families may access service from health care professionals, community agencies, and national organizations. Timely connections with such resources can help reduce feelings of apprehension and isolation.

GETTING HELP FROM HEALTH CARE PROFESSIONALS

Once Parkinson's disease is diagnosed and a family begins the process of accepting this intruder into their lives, many have a "Where Do I Turn?" response. Recently diagnosed patients can begin the quest for knowledge about the disease by seeking information from their physicians. In addition, it is reasonable to request that health care providers arrange contact with another Parkinsonian. Empathic concern from someone who's "been there" can reassure the patient that life with Parkinson's disease will continue to be worthwhile.

Parkinsonians also deserve knowledgeable health professionals to assist them in maintaining optimum health status. At minimum this team should include a neurologist and a primary care physician (family practitioner or internist) to care for general health problems that may coexist with the Parkinson's disease. Some patients may want to consult a movement disorders specialist at a research center from time to time to evaluate the medical regimen and ensure the most up-to-date care.

159

EDUCATIONAL LITERATURE

Helpful educational materials are available to assist a family in making satisfactory adjustments and lifestyle adaptations to live comfortably with this chronic disease. It is important that a recently diagnosed Parkinsonian not be overwhelmed with volumes of literature at the outset. Most patients are better served by their physicians if the latter select one or two brochures to offer at the time of diagnosis; at a second appointment the physician can reassess the patient's understanding of the disease, answer any questions, and provide more in-depth literature if appropriate. Organizations that publish literature targeted to the public and to health professionals interested in Parkinson's disease are listed at the end of this chapter.

SUPPORT GROUP INTERVENTIONS

Parkinson's disease support groups provide a format through which families with common interests and health problems can share their concerns. Many support groups also sponsor ancillary services to aid both patients and caregivers. These may include exercise groups, speech therapy sessions, transportation assistance, and discussion forums for spouses. Both the American Parkinson Disease Association (APDA) and Parkinson's Educational Programs (PEP) sponsor chapters across the country. Independent support groups have also formed in many cities to meet the needs of families coping with Parkinson's disease.

Sometimes people express concern that attending such meetings might be depressing or discouraging. On the contrary, at such meetings new patients typically have an opportunity to visit with fellow Parkinsonians at all disease stages and to recognize that many are managing quite well. A number of participants identify the support group experience as a valued aspect of their lives. Monthly meetings focus on a program, a speaker, or a discussion topic targeted to families who want to learn more about the disease.

COMMUNITY SERVICES

Community agencies provide a variety of services for senior adults that can be particularly helpful to the Parkinsonian whose goal is to continue to manage independent living. Area Agencies on Aging (AAA) sponsor senior citizen centers in most communities in the United States. These centers serve adults over the age of sixty, and offer social, educational, and health-maintenance programs in addition to midday meal service. Most senior centers provide home-delivered meals to participants who are unable to attend the congregate lunch program.

Many senior centers also provide round-trip transportation to the center, to grocery stores, to medical appointments, and for other essential errands. Transportation arrangements vary from scheduled route systems in larger cities to demand/response systems in smaller towns. One of the most frustrating losses Parkinsonians may face as their disease produces increasing limitations is the ability to drive safely. For the person whose spouse is willing and able to take the wheel, this loss may be merely an inconvenience. But for the impaired Parkinsonian who lives alone, being unable to drive constitutes a major handicap. Utilization of the AAA transportation service can help prevent social isolation. Other services offered by such agencies in many locations include:

Information and referral—to assist the public in obtaining help with such matters as social security benefits, food stamps, employment and educational opportunities, health care resources, legal assistance, volunteer opportunities, and shared housing programs;

Adult day care—providing an array of services in a nonresidential setting to dependent older persons who need supervision but not institutionalization;

Legal assistance—to provide aid with such matters as preparing a will, establishing power of attorney, making property decisions, reporting consumer fraud, and understanding their legal rights;

Homebound services—to address special needs regarding household maintenance and assistance with chores, personal care, and telephone reassurance;

Case management—coordination with various community resources to help with complicated or multiple problems such as poor health, limited income, lack of insurance coverage, inadequate housing, and abusive situations;

Elder ombudsmen—who serve as trained advocates for families interacting with hospitals and nursing homes. Parkinsonians unfortunately suffer the same health problems common to other senior adults. The ombudsman can provide assistance with such issues as filing Medicare and other third-party claims or tracking complaints regarding care in long-term care institutions.

Services of the Area Agencies on Aging, federally funded under Title III of the Older Americans Act, are available to all persons over sixty years of age.

INTERMEDIATE CARE OPTIONS

Licensed home health agencies are another important community resource for the Parkinsonian who needs professional nursing or attendant care following an acute illness. Medicare may cover these expenses for varying periods of time when home health services are ordered by a physician. Home health care can be a useful adjunct to shorter hospital stays, helping ensure that patients are not prematurely "on their own" after a major illness. Specific services include skilled nursing procedures, training family members to assume less technical functions, and health aide visits to help with routine tasks such as bathing or feeding the bedfast patient. Once a physician makes the home health referral, a registered nurse performs an initial assessment of each patient and makes recommendations to the family and to the referring physician regarding a comprehensive care plan. Home health services often include social work consultation, physical and occupational therapy, and speech therapy. Agency personnel can recommend and make arrangements to secure durable medical equipment to simplify care at home.

Adult day care centers fulfill a variety of needs for advanced-stage Parkinsonians who live with their families but cannot safely stay alone at home. Such facilities can be lifesavers for primary caregivers, who may themselves be elderly or whose health may also be fragile. Participants in day care programs may attend the center for a varying number of days per week at a daily rate that is more affordable that hourly attendant rates offered by home health agencies. Day care enables the spouses or other family caregivers to accomplish necessary errands and regain sufficient stamina to continue their caregiving obligations. In some cases, the availability of day care for elders provides the caregiver of a Parkinsonian patient the opportunity to continue working.

RESIDENTIAL CARE

While the majority of Parkinsonians never require institutionalized care, approximately one in five do live for some period of time in a long-term care facility. Although there is a trend toward developing retirement centers and foster living arrangements for patients who can no longer live at home, most people who need residential care still utilize the services of traditional nursing homes.

It is crucial for family members to know what factors to look for when selecting a suitable facility for the patient with Parkinson's disease. The following criteria are intended to serve as guidelines to help families identify reputable long-term care centers:

1. Both the facility and the administrator should have a current license from the state. Ask to spend time with the administrator and the director of nursing services to discuss the needs of your relative as a prospective resident in their facility. The facility should have a registered nurse on duty twenty-four hours per day.

2. Cleanliness is a good indicator of the level of care in other areas. Inspect kitchen and bathroom areas. Food on the dining room floor is inevitable at mealtimes, but should not remain two hours later.

3. Casually note the condition of clothing and the gooming of residents. Disarrayed or soiled clothing can be a clue to poor nursing standards or understaffing.

4. Visit a facility unannounced, at different times of day and night. Observe how promptly the nursing staff responds to patient call lights and other requests for help. Since incontinence is a problem for many nursing home residents, an area may have a faint odor on occasion. However, any strong or constant odor of urine or feces should warn a family away from that facility.

5. The physical plant should be pleasant and relatively quiet. Parkinsonians need wide hallways with hand rails along the walls, and bathrooms that are easily accessible. Families need a visiting place away from roommates and communal dining areas.

6. Inquire about patient-to-staff ratios and personnel turnover rates. The best facilities have nurses and aides who genuinely enjoy working with older adults and are able to retain good employees for longer periods of time. It is also worthwhile to inquire if the consulting physician

for a facility has experience with Parkinson's disease, or to make sure the patient's personal physician is willing to continue caring for him or her as a resident of the nursing home.

The nursing home experience can be more positive than imagined by many patients and family members. Primary caregivers can still remain involved in the care of their spouses or parents by providing care on weekends and holidays, spending quality time with their loved ones in their new "home," and keeping watch to ensure that the level of care received remains high. Families and first-rate nursing homes become collaborators to meet the special needs of advanced-stage Parkinsonians.

NATIONAL ORGANIZATIONS

Several national organizations publish excellent educational literature for laypersons and health professionals. One excellent source of information is the American Parkinson Disease Association (APDA). The APDA supplies booklets describing the diagnosis and treatment of Parkinson's disease, exercise instructions, advice about speech and swallowing problems, and assistive devices. In addition to distributing literature, the APDA funds medical research, establishes family support groups, and sponsors thirty-three Parkinson's Disease Information and Referral Centers across the United States. These centers are staffed by neurologists, nurses, and social workers who have special expertise in Parkinson's disease. Services provided include coordinating physician referrals, conducting regional educational conferences, and providing research updates. Many also maintain libraries that loan print and audiovisual materials at no charge.

Another good resource is Parkinson's Educational Programs (PEP), which provides brochures, books, and audiovisual programs at nominal cost to community groups and individuals, in addition to sponsoring affiliated support groups in many locations. Contact information for these and other national organizations is provided at the end of this chapter.

TRAVEL

For the Parkinsonian with sufficient mobility and stamina to enjoy travel, many options exist to make the experience safe and comfortable. For instance, while the aid of a cane or wheelchair may not be necessary in familiar environments, such assistive devices can conserve energy and simplify movement through long airport corridors and busy terminals. A cane can be attractive as well as practical, and can be used to "point balance" through narrow or crowded passageways or even to aid in self-defense should such an unfortunate need arise. Walking canes also carry a subtle message signaling that an altered gait or balance problem is due to a health condition and not intoxication.

Packing lighter and limiting carry-on baggage can also make life easier for the traveler. Physically challenged passengers should take advantage of the preboarding opportunities on scheduled airline flights: do not feel timid about letting airline personnel know of special needs.

It is helpful for the traveling Parkinsonian to carry a letter from a physician, briefly describing any pertinent diagnoses and including a list of prescription medications. This simple document can forestall problems at customs when traveling abroad. Medications should always be kept with the patient rather than being packed in luggage to be checked.

Stephen Birnbaum, noted American travel advisor and author, comments that the travel industry has dramatically improved services to the handicapped in recent years. His books recommend the following access guides to tourist facilities that cater to individuals with physical limitations:

Access to the World, by Louise Weiss (Facts on File, $14.95) This is an excellent guide to handicapped travel, with airport access information.

Frommer's Guide for the Disabled Traveler: The United States, Canada and Europe, by Frances Barish (Simon & Schuster, $10.95). A sightseeing and access guide to seven of the most frequently visited cities in the continental United States, plus Hawaii.

Travel Ability, by Lois Reamy (Macmillan, $13.95) gives vast amounts of information on finding tours for handicapped travelers; coping with public transportation; finding accommodations, special equipment, and travel agents.

Handicapped parking permits simplify travel for Parkinsonians closer to home. Application forms can be obtained from the Motor Vehicle Division of any State Highway Department or local county clerk's office, and must be signed by a physician certifying the handicap. The card is then placed on the dashboard of any vehicle occupied by the handicapped individual. Using this permit enables many Parkinsonians to shop and take care of business independently.

While it is essential for Parkinsonians to access vital support services *from* the communities in which they live, it is equally important for them to remain active contributors *to* society. Churches, charitable organizations, and civic groups need mature volunteers to staff ongoing projects. Parkinsonians can influence their communities in many positive ways—from serving on city council committees to organizing public awareness efforts geared toward educating fellow citizens about this disease, which strikes one percent of adults over age fifty.

Continued involvement in meaningful life pursuits is good preventive medicine to guard against chronic discouragement, mental atrophy, and premature decline in functional levels. Parkinsonain families can learn to accept help in meeting their own needs while simultaneously sharing their unique experience with others.

COMMUNITY SUPPORT SYSTEMS

Resources to Aid the Parkinsonian Family:

The American Parkinson Disease Association (APDA)
116 John Street
New York, New York 10038
(800) 232-2732

PEP*USA - Parkinson's Educational Program
1800 Park Newport #302
Newport Beach, California 92660
(800) 344-7872

The Parkinson's Disease Foundation, Inc.
Williams Black Medical Research Building
640–650 W. 168th Street
New York, New York 10032
(212) 923-4700 or (212) 694-3480

National Parkinson Foundation, Inc.
1501 Ninth Avenue, N.W.
Miami, Florida 33136
(800) 327-4545

United Parkinson Foundation
360 W. Superior Street
Chicago, Illinois 60610
(312) 664-2344

Sears Roebuck and Company
4640 Roosevelt Boulevard
Philadelphia, Pennsylvania 19321
(write or call local catalog desk for medical equipment/supplies catalog)

National Rehabilitation Information Center
Catholic University
4407 Eighth St., N.E.
Washington, D.C. 20017
(202) 635-5826

SUGGESTED READING

Dorros, Sidney. *Parkinson's Disease: A Patient's View.* New York: Warner Books, 1985.

Monnot, Michel. *From Rage to Courage.* St. Denis Press, 1988.

Parkinson's Disease Update (a monthly research publication) Leon Sack, Editor/Publisher, P.O. Box 24622, Philadelphia, Pennsylvania 19111.

Stern, Jan Peter. *The Parkinson's Challenge: A Beginner's Guide to A Good Life in the Slow Lane.* Available only by order: P.O. Box 1817, Santa Monica, California 90406.

14

Forming a Successful Support Group: A Guideline

Fred McGarrett

While working on a research project investigating a new drug developed for the treatment of Parkinson's disease, it was necessary to hospitalize twenty patients for several days. During the study, something somewhat unexpected occurred: As the study progressed, the Parkinsonian patients and their families became very involved with each other and spent much of their free time eagerly discussing the disease. It became quite apparent that these individuals and their families had a great need to talk with each other, to discuss their fears, to compare experiences, and to empathize with each other's embarrassment and frustration regarding their illness.

I (Fred McGarrett) had initially been quite reluctant to participate in the study. Once I became involved, however, I gained so much from the interaction with other Parkinsonian patients that I became one of the founders, and the first president, of the West Texas Parkinsonism Society. I had never even talked to another Parkinsonian patient prior to the study, although more than seven years had passed since I had been diagnosed as having the disease. The other patients reported similar feelings of isolation.

The other patients and I, who were in the study, were hungry for knowledge and for someone to listen to us and to share our concerns. We patients had little understanding of what was causing our disorder and little knowledge regarding what to expect in the days ahead. Our spouses were strong and loving caregivers, but the daily responsibilites of caring for their loved ones frequently aroused feelings of frustration, and of guilt for having such feelings. Fear of what might yet come hung like a black cloud over both the caregivers and their spouses.

I was amazed at the emotional strength we demonstrated. We were brave, kind, emotionally responsive people who showed little bitterness toward the discomfort and inconvenience of our disorder. The group was not looking for an opportunity to complain, but for new ways to cope. Perhaps the most important outcome of the study was the development of a very active and successful support group.

The great need for support was evident in the enthusiastic participation of the group and the rapid growth of membership. Within five years the support group had grown from the 21 families who constituted the first chapter of the West Texas Parkinsonism Society to a regional system with over 700 members and seven chapters in the surrounding areas. Our group's experiences are offered in the hope that we may benefit others who recognize the need for a support group, but who may not be certain how to begin. This chapter will also identify the multiple goals and benefits of being an active participant in a Parkinson's disease support group, and encourage other patients and their families to take advantage of or develop a local support group of their own.

THE PURPOSE OF THE SUPPORT GROUP

The West Texas Parkinsonism Society describes its purpose as follows:

A. To provide assistance to Parkinsonian patients and their families:

   1. By providing accurate information on Parkinsonism through lectures, publications, and other activities.

   2. By assisting in the development and funding of therapeutic or other programs considered to be of value.

   3. By sponsoring and assisting in the establishment of social events and recreational activities for the enrichment of the lives of Parkinsonian patients.

B. To provide public education and information on Parkinsonism in such a way as to better inform the general public on the nature of the disorder, early warning symptoms, methods of treatment and medical management, current research activity, etc.

C. To cooperate with and assist medical societies, physicians, universities, and other institutions in the conduct of research and special studies leading to improved methods of treatment of Parkinsonism.

WHO CAN FORM A SUPPORT GROUP?

I had once inquired of a physician about the advisability of beginning a local support group, but was discouraged by the well-meaning doctor because I only had early symptoms of Parkinson's disease. The physician believed that a person must first show the symptoms to be able to create interest and support for the groups. His viewpoint was obviously wrong. All that is needed to form a support group is a few dedicated people who see the need to bring together patients, families, and other interested people to develop an understanding of Parkinson's disease and to develop successful coping skills.

INITIAL ORGANIZATION OF A SUPPORT GROUP

Although at first the meetings can be held in someone's kitchen over a cup of coffee, soon there will be a need for a comfortable room where meetings can take place according to a regular schedule. To find a suitable place to meet contact banks, churches, senior citizen centers, hospitals, or colleges. These organizations frequently provide space for such organizations free of charge. The West Texas Parkinsonism Society meets regularly in a large classroom at the Texas Tech Health Sciences Center. This has been an ideal setting in that it provides an educational environment with amplifiers, VCRs, overhead projectors, and other audiovisual equipment to assist with presentations.

The West Texas group contacted the American Parkinson Disease Association to request guidance and information on developing a support group. The national association was very helpful in recommending organizational structure and sent sample bylaws for the group to consider. A copy of the West Texas Parkinsonism Society bylaws can be found at the end of this chapter (see Appendix 1).

One of the most important, though sometimes difficult, tasks is to find enthusiastic and energetic individuals who *can* and *will* serve as officers. Initial organization may be a time consuming and demanding task; considerable effort from all interested individuals will be needed to get the program rolling. Requesting additional assistance from professionals in the surrounding community who may have organizational experience and can provide constructive ideas on program planning or are aware of community resources is recommended. The West Texas Parkinsonism Society immediately set up a medical advisory board whose members included neurologists working extensively with Parkinson's disease, as well as clinical psychologists. These directors were invaluable in suggesting activities and providing resources for education. Health professionals who should be considered when developing a board of directors include neurologists, neurosurgeons, psychiatrists, nursing professionals, social workers, speech therapists, physical therapists, etc. The greatest need is to find a neurologist who works with the aged and is interested in the research and clinical aspects of Parkinson's disease. The basic organization of a chapter might consist of a president, vice president, secretary, and treasurer, plus five to seven board members.

Because support groups generally collect dues and donations, a nonprofit status must be established. This can be accomplished by filing the necessary paperwork, which can be obtained from the federal and state governments or by affiliating with a national organization that automatically provides coverage. The membership dues in the Parkinson's Disease Society are kept low to ensure that no one is denied the benefit of the support group because they lack funds. Dues are needed, however, to cover the expenses of maintaining the organization.

PUBLICITY

To increase membership and to advise members of meeting dates and coming events, support group leaders will need to become knowledgeable in providing information to the media. A visit to the library may provide names and addresses of all the newspapers in the territory to be covered. The same can be done with churches.

Most newspapers require that information for publication be submitted two weeks prior to the expected date of appearance in the paper. When mailing the public announcement to the media source, identify date, time, location, and program. Other media such as radio and television can be used for getting special event information out, but they are generally not effective in getting routine monthly meeting information out to the public.

One of the outgrowths of the West Texas support group was the development of a monthly newsletter that was mailed to group members. The newsletter was important for describing upcoming events, but was also an important source of information regarding Parkinson's disease. Not all members will be able to attend each meeting. The newsletter may be the only way they can keep abreast of research efforts and funding. A sample newletter can be found in Appendix 2 of this chapter.

Stuffing and addressing letters is a major undertaking, depending on the size of the group. The effort can be minimized if group members share the responsibility and if enough members meet at one time to complete the job.

MEETINGS

Planning interesting and informative meetings is a challenge to the group's creativity. When planning programs the goals are:

1. to learn about the disease itself and current Parkinson's disease research information;

2. to learn how to better care for ourselves physically and emotionally;

3. to learn about community resources that may not be readily apparent to members;

4. to share common experiences and to support the continued growth of each member;

5. to socialize and, in so doing, reduce social withdrawal and isolation;

6. to develop political awareness and to promote legislation that supports Parkinson's disease research and treatment;

7. to raise funds to support Parkinson's disease research.

Some sample program topics that might be considered are:

TOPIC	SPEAKER
Current status of Parkinson's disease research	neurologist, neurosurgeon
Drug therapy issues	pharmacist, physician
Coping with stress	mental health professional
Home safety	home economist, visiting nurse
Nursing home considerations	nursing home administrator
Legal issues, living wills	attorney
Financial planning	financial planner
Resolving family issues	family therapist
Exercise to maintain health	physical therapist
Speech enhancement	speech therapist
Learning new leisure activities	occupational therapist
Special needs of the spouse	mental health professional
Treatment for depression	psychiatrist, psychologist
Sleep disturbance	psychiatrist, psychologist, neurologist
Understanding Medicare, Medicaid, veteran's benefits	area medicare personnel, veterans administration representative
Access special services for the aged and neurologically handicapped	area Agency on Aging Administrator
Visiting nurse services	visiting nurse personnel

Again, make use of the professionals in your community to provide lectures or demonstrations for your monthly meetings.

Remember, a major goal of the support group is for members to have an opportunity to talk to one another and to support one another. If your group becomes large, periodic small group discussions may be advisable to encourage active participation and to increase feelings of familiarity and comfort. Resist the temptation to overplan your meeting. Seek out a mental health professional to facilitate and encourage a discussion of feelings, fears, and family stresses. A few thought-provoking questions may be all you need to provide a valuable group experience.

Meetings will typically last between one and two hours. Since this is a very long period for Parkinsonian patients to sit in one spot, a refreshment break at the midpoint of the meeting will encourage social interaction and provide an opportunity to stretch weary legs.

The following is a list of activities that may enhance support group monthly meetings:

1. A telephone committee to call members may effectively increase attendance. A friendly call may help show members how important they are to the group. Increased social activity may also result.

2. Assigning members to "greet" those attending makes people feel welcome.

3. Name tags also facilitate discussion and mutual support.

4. Names and addresses of first-time visitors should be taken and added to the mailing list.

5. Refreshments are recommended. In the West Texas society, group members volunteer to bring refreshments. This responsibility is rotated among members.

6. Provide pickup and return for individuals who would like to attend the meeting but are unable to do so on their own.

Forming traditions is a useful way to enhance group cohesion and to provide members with pleasant anticipation. Our society established an annual banquet to honor the "Man or Woman of the Year" who had most significantly contributed to the success of the support group. Individuals who have been honored include physicians, politicians, and people who have worked to promote the well-being of Parkinson's disease patients. The banquet is traditionally held in April in conjunction with Parkinsonian Awareness Week. This banquet provides a good opportunity to encourage public recognition and education regarding Parkinson's disease. Other regularly scheduled social events of our organization include a summer picnic and a Christmas party pot lock supper.

RESEARCH PARTICIPATION

An initial research project brought many of the Parkinsonian patients in our group together. Since then, society members have participated in multiple research projects at the Texas Tech University Health Sciences Center. We believe this to be a very important way to contribute to the understanding of Parkinson's disease and ultimately to enhance treatment and the likelihood of an eventual cure. Through research projects completed in our area and others across the country, a slow-release Sinemet has been developed and will soon be on the market. This new drug may provide more durable relief from Parkinson's symptoms and reduce the on-and-off effect. We take great pride in knowing that the many needle pricks we endured may lead to less suffering of our peers and a greater understanding of our disease. Being involved in research provides a sense of "doing something" about the disease and leaves a feeling of being more in control. Participation in research is sometimes tiring and uncomfortable, but generally it is an interesting and educational experience that supports comradery and provides social experiences.

Research and support are considered so important by our society that in 1985 we provided a one-thousand dollar research grant to be used to develop a motor lab in the Department of Medical and Surgical Neurology at Texas Tech University Medical School. In 1986, we established a three-hundred dollar scholarship award to be given each year to a deserving medical student.

FUND RAISING AND ADVOCACY

Fund raising is not, nor will it ever be, the primary purpose of the support group. Nevertheless, it is an activity in which groups will need to become more experienced and to which more attention will need to be devoted. Fund raising is necessary if the research effort throughout the country is to continue and expand.

Becoming affiliated with a national organization provides local support groups with the benefits of that organization's experiences and resources. Support groups that work together have greater political strength. The pooling of their funds results in improved quality of research as well as expanding the research effort. A list of national organizations and their addresses can be found at the end of chapter 13.

CONCLUSION

When I was first asked to participate in the initial research study I was one of the most difficult to convince that such involvement would benefit me or anyone else. But soon I experienced the relief of sharing my fears and anxieties, the power that knowledge of one's disease can bring, and the satisfaction of supporting others who have similar paths to follow. I have touched many lives, and those whom I touch reach out to still more Parkinsonians and family members. This results in a large, energized, and hopeful community of activity and friendship.

Although the initial organization of the group required much effort, dedication, and diligence in overcoming fears of failure, the support group members take much pleasure and pride in their organization and its accomplishments. Since the first meeting, leadership has changed hands several times and new groups have been formed. The work continues. It requires the participation and sharing of many, but few complain. As I frequently tell new members, "I discovered that I was not alone!"

Appendix 1

Bylaws of the West Texas Parkinsonism Society

ARTICLE I: NAME

The legal name of this organization shall be the West Texas Parkinsonism Society.

ARTICLE II: PURPOSES

The purposes of the West Texas Parkinsonism Society are:

A. To provide assistance to Parkinsonian patients and their families.

   1. By providing accurate information on Parkinsonism through lectures, publications, and other educational activities;

   2. By assisting in the development and funding of therapeutic or other programs considered by the board to be of value;

   3. By sponsoring and assisting in the establishment of social events and recreational activities for the enrichment of the lives of Parkinsonian patients;

   4. By assisting families of Parkinsonian patients in adjusting to the social and functional problems associated with the disorder.

B. To provide public education and information on Parkinsonism in such a way as to better inform the general public on the nature of the disorder, early warning symptoms, methods of treatment and medical management, current research activity, etc.

C. To cooperate with and assist medical societies, physicians, universities, and other institutions in the conduct of research and special studies leading to improved methods of treatment of Parkinsonism.

ARTICLE III: MEMBERSHIP

Section 1. Eligible applicants may obtain membership on application to the Chairman of the Membership Committee:

Section 2. Memberships shall be classified as follows:

A. Family (Patient and Spouse)	$15.00
B. Single	$10.00
C. Supporting	$15.00
D. Donor	

ARTICLE IV: DUES

Section 1. Dues are payable yearly.

Section 2. Dues may be waived by the Board of Directors when the payment would constitute a hardship. Such waiver shall require a simple majority vote of those Directors present.

ARTICLE V: MEETINGS

Section 1. Regular meetings shall be held at least quarterly but may be held monthly by giving two weeks notice in advance of the special meeting. Special meetings may be called by the President on written application to ten members or a majority of the Directors. Requests for a special meeting must state the reason for such special meeting.

Section 2. A quorum shall consist of either 10 percent of the membership or ten members, whichever is greater. They must be present in person.

Section 3. The annual meeting will be held in January of each year.

Section 4. Order of Business

    A. Call to order

    B. Minutes of previous meeting

    C. Treasurer's report

    D. Report of standing committees

    E. Report of special committees

    F. Unfinished business

    G. Secretary's correspondence

    H. New business

    I. Elections (when necessary)

    J. Adjournment

ARTICLE VI: FISCAL YEAR

The fiscal year shall begin January 1 and end December 31 of each year.

ARTICLE VII: BOARD OF DIRECTORS

Section 1. The Board of Directors shall consist of no less than three and no more than seven members elected for a period of three years, one-third elected each year by the members of the Society in regular meeting.

Section 2. The Board of Directors shall be responsible for the conduct of the business of the Society and shall be empowered to employ such professional personnel as required to administer the affairs of the Society and to prescribe their duties. The Board of Directors shall exercise all other powers inherent in the Society except those expressly reserved to the members.

Section 2.1. No director or officer of W.T.P.A. shall have the authority to contract a debt, or incur an obligation on behalf of W.T.P.A. in excess of $200.00 without prior approval of the Board of Directors, unless such item was a part of the Board approved budget. The Board may require bonding of its officers or employees at any time deemed feasible by the Board.

ARTICLE VIII: DUTIES OF THE OFFICERS

Section 1. The President shall preside at all meetings of the membership. All Committee Chairmen will report directly to the President or Vice President. The President shall present an Annual Report of the activities for the year to the members at the Annual Meeting. He shall perform such other duties as prescribed by the Board of Directors.

Section 2. The Vice President shall be responsible to the President. He will perform the duties of the President in the absence of the President. He will perform other duties as may be assigned to him by the President.

Section 3. The Secretary shall maintain a record of all members. He shall maintain a record of all meetings of the members, and of the Board of Directors.

Section 4. The Treasurer shall maintain a complete record of funds received and disbursed. He shall deposit and disburse all funds. The Treasurer and/or any other officer may be empowered by the Board to sign checks for the corporation.

ARTICLE IX: ELECTIONS

Section 1. There shall be a Nominating Committee appointed by the Board of Directors composed of a Chairman and four members. Two and only two of the members of this committee shall be members of the Board of Directors.

Section 2. The Nominating Committee shall prepare a slate of candidates for the election of the President, Vice President, Secretary, Treasurer and Board of Directors and shall secure the consent of each to serve if elected. The Nominating Committee Chairman shall report its nominations to the President or Vice President at least one week prior to the Annual Meeting.

ARTICLE X: PARLIAMENTARY AUTHORITY

Roberts' Rules of Order shall govern the conduct of business in all cases in which they are applicable and not in conflict with the constitution.

The rules of order may be suspended by a two-thirds majority vote of all those present and eligible to vote.

ARTICLE XI: AMENDMENTS

Any proposed amendment, along with the date it is to be voted upon, shall be presented in writing to the entire membership at least two weeks prior to the meeting at which it is to be voted upon; two-thirds majority of those present shall be required for ratification.

Appendix 2

West Texas Parkinsonism Society
and APDA Information Referral Center

NOVEMBER MEETING NEWS:

Thursday, November 6th, 7 P.M. TTUHSC Building, 4th and Indiana, Lubbock, Texas

Program:
   "Fraternity Adoption Plan" by Paul Novak, President Sigma Phi Epsilon, TTU
   Come hear this young man introduce his fraternity to us and hear their plans for working with West Texas Parkinsonism Society next year!

   Officers will also be nominated . . . We *need* your input and presence.

DECEMBER CHRISTMAS DINNER!!

Mark calendars now before the holiday schedule rush begins for our annual WTPS Christmas pot-luck supper. Saturday, December 6th, 6:30 P.M.

   Place: Arnett House—LCC Campus, 22nd and Dover (West of Chicago). *Call: 743-2647 to let us know you're planning to be there!* Turkey, dressing, and ham will be furnished by the Crowders and the Behners!

THE PRESIDENT'S CORNER . . .

The conference in Bermuda was fun—expensive—and *very* educational! I feel so grateful for the opportunity to meet top neurologists and hear the latest updates. Dr. Roger Duvoisin (author of the guidebook for patients and families) and Dr. David Marsden, from the University of London, were my favorites. Marsden indicated the fetal transplant on humans was coming in the near future.

Please fill out the yellow "Involvement Survey" handed out at our last meeting and bring those to the November meeting. I am working like crazy on the Sept./1987 cruise, so please think ahead about the possibility of going on the Parkinson Alaska cruise. More details will be printed soon.

I am so involved with the national mission of APDA that I NEED your help on many levels locally. We do not all have equal talents, but there is something special that each of us can do! Let me know how you think *you* might best serve our chapter and do something good for yourself at the same time.

SMILE . . .God loves you and the CURE is coming!

—Ava—

APDA AWARDS $25,000 TO TECH

The Department of Medical and Surgical Neurology at TTUHSC has been funded for the second consecutive year by the American Parkinson Disease Association to manage a Parkinson's Disease Information and Referral Center in Lubbock.

Fred McGarrett and Ava Crowder, representatives of the area APDA chapter, presented the award check to J. Thomas Hutton, M.D., Director of the IRC, at a press conference earlier this fall.

The grant money is used to pay the coordinator's salary (Hutton volunteers his services as Director of the center), institutional overhead charges, printing and postage costs for area support groups, telephone communications, and routine maintenance and operations expenses of the Information and Referral Center office in the medical school.

The IRC budget is extremely limited in proportion to the goals set for the center, according to Hutton. He stated that efforts are currently in progress to expand the funding base on both national and local levels to secure the monies necessary to continue starting new support groups and otherwise expand services to area families.

Dr. Hutton further commented that he and his department appreciate the history of cooperation and support from the West Texas Parkinsonism Society, and look forward to an ongoing association throughout 1987.

PARKINSON PARTNERS MEETING AGAIN

Approximately 10 spouses of Parkinsonian patients have been meeting this fall at a local church on a regular basis. Susan Imke, R.N., M.S., acts as facilitator for the group, which meets for 1½ hours every other Friday afternoon. Both men and women are welcome to join the group. The only thing that is sometimes more difficult than *being* a Parkinsonian is being married to one!

Call if you'd like to join the group. There is no charge for participation.

VOLUNTEERS STILL NEEDED IN THE INFORMATION AND REFERRAL CENTER TO WORK 3 HOURS PER WEEK. CALL FOR MORE DETAILS . . . .

Newsletter Format to be Revised:

In order to reduce the printing and postage costs of mailing monthly newsletters to separate support groups in Lubbock and Amarillo, the Information and Referral Center will be publishing a combined newsletter starting January, 1987.

The publication will be sponsored by the TTUHSC Information and Referral Center and will include meeting announcements for all area support groups. There will be a combined issue in November and December, and a combined issue during the summer months. All other issues will continue to come out monthly.

All officers, board members, and support group members are encouraged to submit articles to be included in the newsletters.

DRUG UPDATE:

Medication: *Disipal* (generic name: orphenadrine hydrochloride) . . . demonstrates parasympatholytic and *anti-tremor* activity; the drug acts centrally, producing effective relaxation of muscle activity . . . produces less drowsiness than other drugs in its class.

Dosage: 50 mg. two or three times daily

Side Effects: dry mouth; rarely causes heart palpitations; avoid using Darvon in combination with Disipal.

BATHROOM SAFETY EQUIPMENT AND GROOMING AIDS

Safety is essential in the bathroom; it is probably the most dangerous room in the average house for anyone who has impaired balance, difficulty walking, tremor, or decreased voice volume.

A tile floor can be slippery, and the surfaces of the shower or tub are extremely slippery when wet. Often the room is small and offers restricted walking space. A call for help may go unheard, especially if water is running in the tub or lavatory. Adequate equipment and an awareness of safety factors increase the ease of bathing and grooming without mishap . . . .

1. Soap on a rope keeps soap conveniently within reach while showering or taking a tub bath.

2. A suction brush, for nail care, and a soap dish can be attached to the inside of the tub, shower, or sink.

3. A sponge attached to a long handle, or a soft, long-handled bath brush will reach the lower legs, feet, and back. They help eliminate bending and are necessary if you have a problem with balance.

4. Wash mitts or terry cloth gloves that eliminate the need for washcloths.

5. An electric razor should be used for safety, particularly if you have Parkinson's tremor. A variety of electric razor holders are commercially available to make it easier for you to grasp the razor.

6. Glass tumblers should not be used in the bathroom if you have difficulty holding objects. Paper or plastic cups are safe, inexpensive, and disposable.

7. Nonskid decorative decals or strips should be attached to the tub or shower floor, or rubber mats placed on these surfaces; these are essential to help eliminate falls. Small bathroom rugs are easily

tripped over and should not be used on the floor if you have difficulty walking. Use a large rug that covers most of the floor; wall-to-wall carpeting; or bare, unwaxed flooring.

8. Tub seats or shower chairs make showering easier and safer. An inexpensive, flexible shower hose that can reach the seated person may be attached to the shower head. A shower nozzle with a turn-off knob is more convenient than a free-flow nozzle.

9. Grab bars should be placed in strategic locations around the tub or shower. Never put weight on towel racks or soap holders affixed to the wall; they were not designed as grab bars and may break away under pressure.

10. A raised toilet seat makes sitting on and rising from the toilet easier. Arm rails attached to the toilet, or a grab bar installed on the wall adjacent to the toilet, provide convenient hand holds.

11. A night light should always be installed in a wall socket in the bathroom.

Glossary

Acetylcholine: one of the major chemicals in the brain, see **Neurotransmitter**

Agnosia: inability to hear, see, or perceive even though the sensory systems are functioning and intact

Akinesia: complete or partial loss of muscle movement

Amantadine (hydrochloride): a medication initially designed to relieve influenza symptoms but later found to help rigidity, slowness of movement, and tremor in Parkinsonism

Anticholinergic agents: substances (medications) that adversely affect nerve endings that allow the chemical acetylcholine to be emitted

Antihistaminic medication: drugs designed to reduce the natural histamine level, which increases when certain tissues of the body are injured or irritated; they appear to have other properties that inhibit production of acetylcholine

Antioxidant: agent that prevents the loss of oxygen (oxidation) in chemical reactions

Aphasia: inability to express oneself through speech

Apraxia: inability to act in a purposeful way even though capable of moving and comprehending

Arteriosclerotic: resulting from hardened arteries

Aspiration: the labored sucking of air

Aspiration pneumonia: pneumonia that occurs after having breathed foreign matter into the lungs

Autonomic nervous system: nervous system that serves the involuntary body functions (e.g., breathing, the beating of the heart)

Basal ganglia: deep structures of the brain

Benzodiazepine: a class of transquilizers, which includes diazepam (Valium), chlordiazepoxide (Librium), and alprazolam (Xanax), which do not result in Parkinsonism or Parkinson-like symptoms.

187

Bilateral: occurring on both sides of the body (left and right)

Blepharospasm: rapid blinking or forced closure of the eyes

Blood pressure cuff: the part of the instrument used for measuring blood pressure that is wrapped around the upper arm

Bradykinesia: slow or reduced movement

Cadence: rhythm of measured movement

Chlorpromazine (Thorazine): a transquilizing medication that can cause Parkinson-like symptoms

Cholinergic system: system of nerve endings that permit the emission of the chemical acetylcholine

Clonazepam: medication to relieve sudden muscle spasms (see **Nocturnal myoclonus**)

Cognition: awareness; having perception and memory

Cogwheeling (also known as lead pipe rigidity): regular, slow, jerking movements; often associated with the tremors that accompany Parkinson's disease

Condom catheter: a condom-like apparatus that fits over the penis in a manner that permits emptying of the bladder into a bag connected to the catheter with tubing

Corpus striatum: a vital part of the brain, located beneath the cerebral cortex (outer covering of the brain) and comprised of two basal ganglia (caudate and putamen)

Cyclotron: instrument used to smash electrons thereby emitting energy for analysis

Delirium: disorientation with respect to time and place, often accompanied by illusions and hallucination; a state of mental confusion/excitement

Dementia: progressive deterioration of mental state

Demerol: an addictive pain medication

Distended abdomen: stretched or inflated

Dopamine: a chemical produced by the brain; it assists in the effective transmission of electrochemical messages between neurons (see **Neurotransmitter**)

Dyskinesia: abnormal movement of voluntary muscles (e.g., in the hand, arm, leg, etc.)

Encephalitis: inflammation of the brain

Endocrine disorders: diseases or dysfunctions of any or all of the following glandular network: thyroid, parathyroid, adrenal gland, pituitary (anterior and posterior), testes/ovaries

Essential tremor: a rapid tremor that, in contrast to the slower, resting tremor of Parkinson's disease, increases with limb extension (see **tremor**)

Familial tremor: an inherited essential tremor (see **tremors**)

Fecal impaction: feces wedged in the bowel making elimination very difficult

Festinating gait: rapid, uncontrolled shuffling

Flexion contracture: permanent bending of parts of the body

Fluphenazine (Prolixin): a tranquilizing medication that can cause Parkinson-like symptoms

Glaucoma: increased pressure of the eyeball, which can result in nerve damage and blindness

Haloperidol (Haldol): a tranquilizing medication that can cause Parkinson-like symptoms

Heimlich maneuver: a form of first aid for choke victims

Hypomanic mood: mild excitement with moderate change in behavior

Infused (intravenous): introducing a substance to the body via injection through a vein

Lacunes: small strokes

Loxapine (Loxitane): a transquilizing medication that can cause Parkinson-like symptoms

Metabolism: the assimilation and processing of substances in the body (e.g., transforming food into energy, utilizing vitamin and mineral compounds, etc.)

Motor performance: ability and capacity to move about and to maneuver the body

MPTP (N-methyl-4-phenl-1,2,3,6-tetrahydropyridine): a toxic chemical the use of which can lead to Parkinsonism

Multi-infarct disease: interruption of blood flow, which results in strokes

Muscle atrophy: wasting of muscle tissue due to lack of use as a result of being immobilized or from injury to the nerve that normally stimulates a muscle

Musculoskeletal: the interrelationship of muscles and bone structures

Neurofibrillary tangles: tangles of tiny fibers in nerve cells

Neurotransmitter: chemicals that permit nerve cell communication in the brain

Neurovegetative syndrome: symptoms affacting the involuntary nervous system that controls body functions and glandular secretions

Nocturnal myoclonus: sudden muscle jerks occurring at night

Norepinephrine: see **Neurotransmitter**

Off dystonia: an abnormal posturing or cramping when levodopa levels are at their minimum in the bloodstream (see **Levodopa**)

Oil retention enema: oil injected into the rectum to soften feces to improve elimination

On dystonia: abnormal movement when levodopa levels are at their peak in the bloodstream (usually 20 to 60 minutes after dosage)

Orthostatic hypotension: a drop in blood pressure during rapid changes in body position (e.g., from a sitting position to standing position)

Paroxysmal disorder: sudden onset of a disease or symptom

Perseveration: repeating meaningless statements, phrases, words, or speaking repetitively when it bears no relation to the context

Postencephalitic Parkinsonism: Parkinsonism that results from inflammation and infection of the brain

Preclinical: prior to diagnosis of a disease

Propulsive gait: walking that is propelled forward

Psychomotor agitation: physical activity due to excited state of mind

Psychotic disorder: mental disturbance resulting in loss of personality and loss of contact with reality

Pulmonary emboli: a mass of undissolved matter in the main artery of the lung or one of its branches

Radiolabeled: marking a substance for detection with radiation

Reserpine: a drug prescribed for high blood pressure or as a tranquilizer; its use may give rise to Parkinsonism

Resting tremor: shaking even though the body (or limb) is not being put in motion by the effected individual

Retropulsive gait: walking that is propelled backward

Serotonin: see **Neurotransmitter**

Sialorrhea: drooling

Substantia nigra: black pigmented area of the mid-brain

Toxin: a poisonous substance

Tremor: rhythmic shaking; an involuntary movement of part(s) of the body as a result of sequential muscle contractions

Tremulous voice: trembling or shaking voice

Trifluroperazine (Stelazine): a tranquilizing medication that can cause Parkinson-like symptoms

Voice inflection: change of pitch or tone

Contributors

KATHRYN L. BLAKESLEY, M.A., is a speech language pathologist in private practice in Houston, Texas. She has served as a consultant to the Houston Area Parkinsonism Society and as a diagnostician and speech pathologist with nursing homes and home health care agencies. She has presented numerous workshops in hospitals and nursing homes.

JIM R. CARPENTER, B.S., P.T., is technical director of physical medicine and rehabilitation at St. Elizabeth Hospital, the Kate Dishman Rehabilitation Center and Med-Therapy Outpatient Unit, which provides work-hardening and work-simulation service for industry. These units are all part of the St. Elizabeth Hospital System, which is located in Beaumont, Texas.

NELDA DAVIS DIPPEL, R.N.C., M.S.N., is assistant professor in the School of Nursing at Texas Tech University Health Sciences Center, Lubbock, Texas, where she also serves as Director of the Nursing Center. She is certified by the American Nurses Association as a Gerontological Nurse.

RAYE LYNNE DIPPEL, Ph.D., is a clinical psychologist and life-span developmental psychologist who is currently in private practice in Houston, Texas. She is also a clinical assistant professor of psychiatry and behavioral sciences at the University of Texas Medical School at Houston. She recently coedited (with Dr. J. Thomas Hutton) *Caring for the Alzheimer Patient: A Practical Guide.* Dr. Dippel has presented numerous lectures on aging, dementia, and Parkinson's disease and has published several research articles on these topics.

193

JEFFREY W. ELIAS, Ph.D., is professor and associate chair of the Department of Psychology at Texas Tech University at Lubbock, Texas. His research program has concentrated on the cognitive changes that occur with age and the effects of disease processes on normal aging. Dr. Elias is the experimental studies editor of the journal *Experimental Aging Research*. His recent publications include co-authoring a chapter with Merrill Elias, and P. K. Elias for the recent revision of the *Handbook of the Psychology of Aging*. Dr. Elias is coeditor of the text *Cardiovascular Disease and Behavior*.

J. THOMAS HUTTON, M.D., Ph.D., is professor of medical and surgical neurology at the Texas Tech University Health Sciences Center in Lubbock, Texas. He is also the Director of the Parkinson's Disease Information and Referral Center. Dr. Hutton recently received a resolution from the Texas Senate praising him for his clinical research and organizational activities to benefit older Texans. As a practicing neurologist, he carries out an active research program in Parkinson's disease. Dr. Hutton also has coedited (with A. D. Kenny) *Senile Dementia of the Alzheimer Type;* edited a volume of neurologic clinics entitled *Dementia;* and coedited (with Raye Lynne Dippel, Ph.D.) *Caring for the Alzheimer Patient: A Practical Guide.*

SUSAN IMKE, R.N., M.S., is a certified family nurse practitioner and instructor of neurology at the Texas Tech University Health Sciences Center in Lubbock, Texas, and serves as the coordinator for the Neurology of Aging Information and Referral Center in the School of Medicine. She has extensive experience working with older adults who are coping with chronic health problems, and is currently involved in clinical practice, research, and educational programs for caregivers as well as health professionals interested in Parkinson's disease and Alzheimer's disease.

WILLIAM C. KOLLER, M.D., Ph.D., is professor and chairman of the Department of Neurology at the University of Kansas Medical Center in Kansas City. Dr. Koller is interested in research in Parkinson's disease and tremor disorders. He is on the Board of Directors of the United Parkinson Foundation and is chairman of the International Tremor Foundation. He has published many articles related to movement disorders. Dr. Koller is also editor of *Handbook of Parkinson's Disease* and coeditor of *Therapeutic Approaches to Parkinson's Disease*.

HENRICK K. KULMALA, Ph.D., is assistant editor in biochemistry at the chemical abstracts service in Columbus, Ohio, and former assistant professor of pharmacology at Northeastern Ohio University's College of Medicine in Rootstown. He has conducted basic research in Alzheimer's disease and in Parkinson's disease and has publications in these areas.

CAROLYN E. MARSHALL, M.P.H., is community education coordinator for the South Texas Geriatric Education Center at the University of Texas Health Sciences Center at San Antonio. Mrs. Marshall is the associate director of the American Parkinson's Disease Information and Referral Center at the University of Texas Health Sciences Center. In her position as community education coordinator, she has produced a number of video tapes on health education including the video "Alzheimer Disease through the Eyes of the Caregiver." Mrs. Marshall is also on the Board of Directors of the Alzheimer Disease Family Support Group of San Antonio. Her Master's thesis, "Architectual Design and the Incidence of Falls among the Aging," provided important insight into the serious problem of falls in the aged.

FRED P. McGARRETT is one of the cofounders and the first president of the West Texas Parkinsonism Society in Lubbock, Texas. Mr. McGarrett was diagnosed as having Parkinson's disease in 1975.

TERRY C. McMAHON, M.D., is an associate professor of psychiary and assistant dean for medical education in the School of Medicine at the Texas Tech University Health Sciences Center in Lubbock. As director of the Psychiatric Consultation Liaison Service, and director of Undergraduate Education in Psychiatry, he has played an active role in developing clinical lectures and seminars for medical students and residents in geriatric psychiatry.

MICHEL MONNOT, Ph.D., is a professor at Carleton College in Northfield, Minnesota, with a research specialty in phonetics. He has been interested in the development of Parkinson's disease since he was diagnosed as having the disease in 1982. Since that time Dr. Monnot has been an active participant in APDA support groups and has become a spokesman for the organization. He received national recognition in 1986 when he walked from Minneapolis to Los Angeles, raising over $400,000 for APDA and resulting in the creation of fourteen new support groups. The APDA Monnot Walkathon was created in his honor and has been a yearly event that has raised nearly $1,000,000 this year alone to fund Parkinson's disease research and to provide support services for individuals who have the disease. In 1988, he authored *From Rage to Courage,* which has been an inspiration to thousands of patients and caregivers.

FRANK L. WILLIAMS is the executive director of the American Parkinson Disease Association. He developed Operation Outreach, which is geared to educating the Parkinsonian community through symposiums and seminars, and the development of information and referral services as well as chapters and support groups. APDA is currently active in forty-eight states, providing patient services, education, and support to thousands of Parkinsonians.

KAREN BOYD WORLEY, Ph.D., is a clinical psychologist in private practice in Little Rock, Arkansas. Dr. Worley specializes in family therapy.